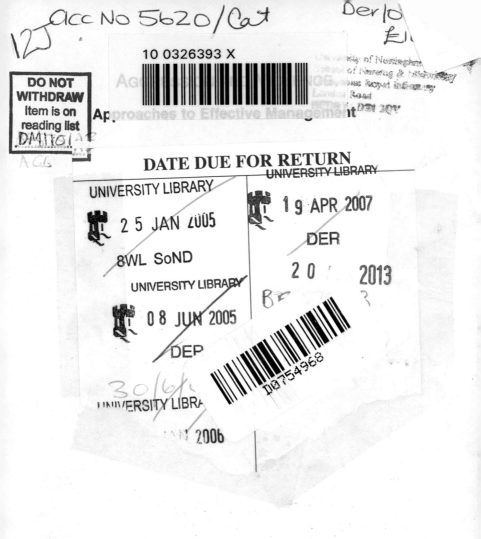

AGGRESSION AND VIOLENCE

Approaches to Effective Management

Edited by
John Turnbull and Brodie Paterson

MACMILLAN

First published 1999 by
MACMILLAN PRESS LTD
Houndmills, Basingstoke, Hampshire RG21 6XS
and London
Companies and representatives throughout the world

ISBN 0–333–62251–0

A catalogue record for this book is available from the British Library.

This book is printed on paper suitable for recycling and made from
fully managed and sustained forest sources.

10 9 8 7 6 5 4 3 2 1
08 07 06 05 04 03 02 01 00 99

Editing and origination by
Aardvark Editorial, Mendham, Suffolk

Printed in Malaysia

To Rhîan, Beci and Rachel

CONTENTS

NOTES ON CONTRIBUTORS

Colin Beacock MA, RNMH, RGN, CertEd was formerly Senior Education Officer at Rampton Hospital and is now a Professional Officer with the Royal College of Nursing. He is also co-editor (with Bob Gates) of *Dimensions of Learning Disability*, published in 1997.

Vaughan Bowie is a Lecturer in the Department of Social Policy and Human Services at the University of Western Sydney. He is the author of *Coping with Violence: A Guide for Human Services* and has been involved in the training of nurses and other health care workers in Australia, Canada, the United States and Northern Ireland.

David Leadbetter MSc, BA(Hons), CQSW, DSW, CSWE is an independent consultant trainer. He has published extensively on issues relating to aggression and violence at work, particularly in health care and social work settings.

Brodie Paterson MEd, BA(Hons), RMN, RNMH, RNT, DipNursing is a Lecturer in the Department of Nursing and Midwifery at the University of Stirling. An experienced trainer and practitioner, he has been involved for many years in research, publication and practice development in the field of managing aggression and violence.

Cheryl Tringham MPhil, RNT, RGN, RNMH is a Teaching Fellow in the Department of Nursing and Midwifery at the University of Stirling. She has a special interest in the professional, legal and ethical issues that arise within health care.

John Turnbull BA, MSc, RNMH is Director of Nursing at Oxfordshire Learning Disability NHS Trust. He has extensive experience as a practitioner, researcher and manager in the field of learning disability and has published widely on a range of topics. His previous post was that of Nursing Officer at the Department of Health.

Rob Wondrak MSc(PsychCouns), BA(Hons), CertEd, RMN, SRN, RNT is Head of Psychosocial Health, Oxford Brookes University, Isis Education Centre, Oxford.

1

INTRODUCTION

John Turnbull and Brodie Paterson

The aim of this book

All the contributors to this book share a common aim of exploring ways in which violence and aggression towards staff in public services can be managed more successfully. They also share with many of the readers of this book the common experience of being victims of violent and aggressive attacks during their careers.

Being assaulted at work is an experience that arouses several different and sometimes conflicting emotions. Even for an experienced professional, fear is the usual initial reaction: fear of further immediate blows or more serious injury, and also anxiety about what others will think of them. Many will feel angry, frequently with themselves because they believe they should have foreseen and thus avoided the incident. Sometimes, they will feel that they have failed or let down colleagues, or that they themselves have been let down by the organisation. Amid all of this, the physical impact of violence seems secondary to its emotional impact, especially while the adrenaline is still pumping around the body following an attack.

This distress can also be made worse if the assailant is well known to the victim. In many instances, they may enjoy a close professional relationship, which makes it difficult for the victim to understand and explain what has happened.

Can violence and aggression be avoided? Where does violence come from? Does training help to reduce the number of incidents? Can the impact of violence be made less traumatic? Whose responsibility is it to ensure that the workplace is safer for employees? This book will explore these questions and many others. Its central aim is to equip readers with knowledge that the authors hope will enable them to cope more successfully with violence and aggression. It draws upon research evidence and the experience of the contributors to explain the dynamics of violence and aggression, and to outline strategies that have been helpful in a variety of settings. The contents place the emphasis on the *management* of violence and aggression rather than its *treatment*. Although some issues will overlap, readers interested in clinical approaches are referred to the growing number of excellent texts on the subject (see Goldstein and Keller 1987, Howells and Hollin 1987).

An occupational hazard?

Throughout this book, violence and aggression will be examined as an occupational rather than a clinical problem. In the same way that organisations have established policies and practices aimed at reducing the risk of back injury or guiding staff in the handling and storing of hazardous substances, the following chapters will unfold evidence and ideas about how violence to staff can be reduced. Although many of the approaches can be transferred to a variety of settings, research would suggest that staff working in the field of health and social services are more vulnerable than others. As a result, much of the research on the subject has been carried out in these settings. Consequently, the text is aimed primarily at front-line staff whose job it is to provide care and support for the public. Those responsible for managing and educating staff, however, will also find its contents useful.

A context for violence and aggression

Before going on to describe the chapters, it is useful to begin by setting violence and aggression in a social, occupational and organisational context and explaining some of the terms that will be used in this book.

Physical harm alone is not sufficient to define a violent incident. For example, someone who accidentally bumps into another person could not be considered to be behaving violently. If the perpetrator had intended to cause harm to the other person, these actions could be described as aggressive, whether or not the victim suffered injury. To give another example, placing an object in a position where there was a good chance of someone tripping over it would be seen as aggression. Where physical injury is suffered and the perpetrator intends to inflict this harm, this would be construed as violence. Thus, aggression is a less precise term that describes a willingness to inflict emotional or physical harm to another, whether or not this is sustained.

In the context of the law, violence is seen simply as the unlawful use of force, which may range from the slightest unwanted contact to homicide. The seriousness of the assault is typically seen by the public as a continuum, with verbal threats at one end of the scale and acts such as rape and murder at the other (Figure 1.1).

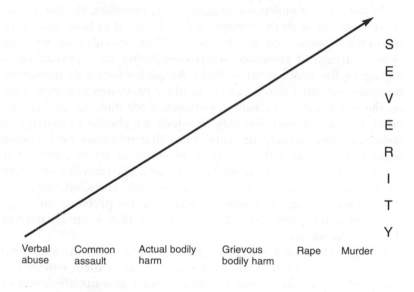

| Verbal abuse | Common assault | Actual bodily harm | Grievous bodily harm | Rape | Murder |

Figure 1.1   Linear model of violence and aggression

In practically all societies, the law exists to establish a set of rules to keep order and to lay down procedures governing the consequences of breaching these rules. If we think about violence and aggression, the law first needs to establish the intention of the suspect. For example, was the person acting in self-defence or did he or she intend to murder his or her victim? Was the person using reasonable force to defend himself or herself when the injury took place? The law might also wish to take into account the circumstances that led up to the incident, for example the degree of provocation that the assailant suffered. Although this might not affect the guilt of the person, it might affect his or her sentence.

To what extent does the law take into account the harm suffered by the victim? As Figure 1.1 shows, our view of the seriousness of an assault is usually governed by our knowledge of the physical harm sustained. However, as this book will show, the emotional impact of another's actions can have more far-reaching conse-quences than any physical injury experienced. For example, staff will often describe the cumulation of threats and verbal abuse as being more distressing than a physical blow. As a manager or colleague, should we take this into account when estimating the risk to staff or the level of support we believe that someone needs?

On the issue of violence and aggression, therefore, the law seems fairly clear cut in its definitions and in the need to take account of the setting conditions for incidents. This provides us with an obvious frame of reference when developing our approaches to managing the problem in services. As professionals or managers, however, we must also be aware of other processes in society that, on the one hand, can create opportunities for violence but, on the other, might influence the way in which we choose to manage it. Societies often develop informal rules that influence how people should think about the lifestyles of some of its members. For example, there is no law against being a new age traveller, although the freedom to pursue this lifestyle is severely curtailed. Similarly, there is no law against having a mental health problem, although this condition is punished in terms of the negative language used to describe the sufferer.

The prejudices of both the users of a service and the staff who work in it are not left at the door when either of them enters. The effects of this could be that violence is seen as a manifestation of someone's condition when, in fact, the person might be expressing anger at having his freedom curtailed or frustration at others' lack of understanding. For example, we might attribute a violent outburst by someone to their learning disability and decide to put up with it. This will serve only to increase the level of violence, which in turn reinforces the view that such people are aggressive. This situation is hardly likely to lead to the successful management of violence. The point is that we must learn to appreciate the role played by our own and others' expectations in generating the potential for violence. This means that we must take a broader view of the causes of violence and see it as a dynamic process; this is illustrated in Figure 1.2.

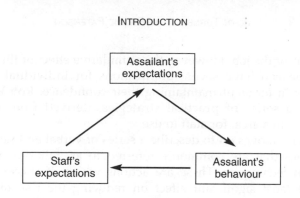

Figure 1.2   Dynamic model of violent and aggressive incidents

Chapter contents

The chapters that follow explore these and many other issues and themes in more detail. Chapter 2 will begin the process of managing the risk to staff by identifying from research evidence the key trends in violence and aggression towards staff. It is difficult for individual staff working day in and day out to gain any perspective on whether their level of fear relates to who they are or where they work. Although some types and grades of staff appear to be more vulnerable than others, the discussion explores the influence of gender, place of work and type of client as well as occupational factors. Once more, it may be that it is an interaction between a number of these factors, rather than a single feature, that generates risk.

Chapter 3 begins the search for more successful management by introducing and discussing the main theories of violence and aggression. Two schools of thinking on the subject, instinctivism and behaviourism, are presented as being the most influential theories in this area; these are compared and contrasted according to their usefulness in providing staff with coping strategies.

Chapter 4 commences a series of chapters examining the strategies that staff can employ to prevent and manage violence and the knowledge they will need to do so. Here, Brodie Paterson and Cheryl Tringham show how essential it is for professionals to have a sound grasp of ethical and legal principles before devising any approach to managing violence. Chapter 5 continues by exploring the problem of verbal abuse, which may be the most common form of aggression encountered by staff. This is something that staff have traditionally regarded as being part of the job. However, the cumulative effect of this type of aggression can have severe implications for individual helpers, especially in terms of maintaining their confidence. Rob Wondrak provides a series of practical strategies, derived from his own research in this area, for staff to use.

Chapter 6 moves on to describe a series of verbal and non-verbal approaches that are commonly referred to as 'talk-down' or de-escalation techniques. These are actions which, if successful, can have the most significant effect on reducing the risk of serious injury to staff and others. Unfortunately, many staff discard their verbal skills as soon as violence occurs. Brodie Paterson and David Leadbetter first point out that de-escalation skills are primarily for use in seeking to reduce a person's arousal, whether or not violence has occurred. Therefore, it is essential that these skills continue to be employed until the person regains control over him or herself. The authors also present one of the first theoretical frameworks for de-escalation to give readers a clearer rationale for their actions.

The use of physical intervention skills in managing violence and aggression is controversial, and Brodie Paterson and David Leadbetter begin Chapter 7 by discussing the main arguments in this area. One of the greatest difficulties in recent times has been the increase in the number of people offering training in physical intervention. This has resulted in a greater variation in the techniques that are taught, but little information for managers on which to judge their comparative effectiveness. The authors, therefore, take an evidence-based approach to this subject and provide some benchmarks against which techniques should be judged.

As this introduction has already pointed out, being a victim of violence and aggression is a distressing experience. Although some staff have developed their own ways of coping over the years, these may not always be the most effective or efficient ways of helping themselves. Furthermore, because violence and aggression are often regarded as clinical problems, organisations rarely initiate programmes aimed at helping their staff to overcome their experience. Therefore, in Chapter 8, Vaughan Bowie calls upon his extensive research and experience in helping victims in different parts of the world to describe some practical approaches to supporting staff.

Education has a major role to play in helping individuals and organisations to manage the problem of violent and dangerous behaviour. The education of professional and non-professional staff is also undergoing a major change at the present time in the United Kingdom. Therefore, in Chapter 9, Colin Beacock takes the opportunity of giving us an overview of the issues in order that staff and managers alike are better able to make choices over the direction for education in this area.

Finally, in Chapter 10, John Turnbull discusses the manager's role in relation to managing risk in services. Here a framework is presented to enable managers, in partnership with their staff, to assess the level of risk in their service and put in place strategies that will enable the service to reduce the incidence of violence and aggression. An important question for managers is how the management of violence can be compatible with the aims of the service and the values held by staff. Using many examples from practice, the author shows how this can be achieved.

References

Goldstein A. and Keller H. (1987) *Aggressive Behaviour: Assessment and Intervention*, Oxford, Pergamon.

Howells K. and Hollin C.R. (eds) (1987) *Clinical Approaches to Violence*, Chichester, John Wiley.

2

VIOLENCE TO STAFF: WHO IS AT RISK?

John Turnbull

Introduction

Violence is a problem that affects people emotionally as well as physically. To understand how we can minimise the risks to staff, we need to begin by looking at which of them are more likely to become victims and in what circumstances. For example, does it make a difference if you are a nurse or a social worker? Are you at greater risk if you are a man or a woman? Are some units or workplaces more dangerous than others? Are there some groups of people for whom you care or support more likely to become violent?

This chapter will seek out answers to such questions. It will not isolate the specific causes of violence: Chapter 3 will discuss the main theoretical approaches to understanding *why* violence occurs. This chapter will instead look at where violence is more likely to happen and to *whom*.

Scanning the evidence

Getting an accurate picture of the scale of violence to staff is fraught with difficulties. Although aggression and violence towards staff is not a new phenomenon, systematic study in this area is a relatively recent phenomenon (Lanza 1983, Lipscombe and Love 1992) and many aspects of violence towards staff remain unexplored. This makes it difficult to confirm the beliefs of some (Castledine 1993, Ryan and Postner 1993) that the problem is growing. Other problems face researchers: as we saw in Chapter 1, concepts such as violence and aggression are not easily defined. Therefore, researchers in the area have tended to use different definitions, making it more difficult to compare results and draw firm conclusions.

Another problem is that most researchers have relied solely upon staff to report violent incidents. We might think that this method is reliable but studies have consistently demonstrated that the majority of assaults go unreported. The degree to which they are unreported is unknown. However, in a key study by Lion *et al.* (1981), it was shown that the actual number of assaults could be as much as five times that of the officially reported incidents. A similar conclusion was drawn by Rowett (1986) in his study of violence to social workers.

It is worth considering why so many incidents go unreported. It may be that some staff are prepared to tolerate a certain level of aggression and will only report the more serious incidents. Another reason might be that staff face so much aggression that they would simply be unable to do their job if they were filling out report forms after every incident. A third reason may be the influence of the organisational culture of a service. If action is not taken by managers following incidents, staff are less likely to report them, which may lead to an acceptance of the inevitability of assaults. Finally, one way in which staff cope with their strong emotions following an incident is to try to change their view of what happened. For example, in Lanza's (1983) study of assaulted nurses, victims said that they believed assailants to be confused at the time or 'not in their right mind'. Thus, if staff believe that their attacker did not intend to hurt them, they are less inclined to record an incident as an assault.

Issues such as these warrant further investigation. In the meantime, we must bear them in mind when interpreting the data from studies on violence.

The Health Services Advisory Committee

We shall begin by looking at a study carried out by the Health Services Advisory Committee (HSAC) on violence to staff in the health service (Health Services Advisory Committee 1987). This study remains the largest of its kind so deserves special mention in a book on violence.

The HSAC survey aimed to assess the severity and extent of violence to staff in five Area Health Authorities in England. One thousand questionnaires were distributed to each Health Authority for further distribution to a range of staff. The questionnaire asked staff to give details of their experiences of violent incidents in the previous 12 months.

Incidents were categorised according to the following criteria:

- **Major incident:** incident resulting in medical assistance
- **Minor incident:** incident resulting in first aid
- **Weapon:** incidents involving a threat with a weapon
- **Verbal abuse:** incidents in which the victim was the object of verbal abuse or threats.

(Adapted from HSAC 1987, p. 1)

Three thousand questionnaires were returned, representing 60 per cent of those distributed. This, claim the authors, was sufficient for the survey to be considered representative of the whole of the National Health Service (NHS).

The results for different hospitals or locations, as well as the severity of the incidents, are shown in Table 2.1.

Table 2.1 Experience of violent incidents classified by hospital type or location and by severity

	Major	Minor	Weapon	Threat
Children's	0.7	9.2	1.3	13.8
General	0.2	9.3	4.6	17.9
Older people's	0.6	21.3	3.9	15.2
Maternity	0	3.8	1.1	8.7
Learning disability	2.0	20.9	7.1	19.9
Mental health	1.6	26.8	11.8	30.7
Community	0.2	3.3	3.9	18.7

Prevalence rates expressed as a percentage of those responding from each location.
Source: Adapted from HSAC 1987, p. 2.

In practical terms, these figures tell a story of 15 staff each year who are involved in a major violent incident. Additional information obtained during the HSAC survey showed that over one-third of these staff needed to take 3 or more days off work. Comparisons with other occupational groups are difficult to make because organisations will define violence in slightly different ways. However, the HSAC offers information for comparison from Home Office studies for England and Wales into violence towards police officers. This shows that staff in the health service are 10 times more likely to be victims of a major physical assault. In her review of similar statistics, Breakwell (1989, p. 29) estimates that health service staff are 26 times more likely to suffer serious injury than the general public. She goes on to conclude that the rate of serious injury in the health service is twice that of the construction industry and five times that of the manufacturing sector. Whether or not Breakwell's estimates are accurate, the point is that health service staff are at significant risk.

Returning to the figures in Table 2.1, we can see clear differences between the risks faced by staff working in different settings. The issue, then, is whether these variations can be accounted for by the characteristics of the staff, the people they care for, a combination of the two or some other factor. These factors will now be discussed in turn.

Occupational factors

Nurses

Using the information from the HSAC survey, Table 2.2 suggests that nurses are the group of health service workers who are at greatest risk of assault.

Table 2.2 Prevalence of violent incidents classified by selected occupational groups and by severity

	Major	Minor	Weapon	Threat
Hospital doctors	0.5	5.9	3.0	19.3
General practitioners	0.5	0.5	5.0	24.9
Student nurses	1.6	36.4	13.6	40.2
Staff nurse	0	20.2	7.3	33.7
Charge nurse	1.6	17.2	8.6	24.2
Ambulance staff	1.7	17.4	17.4	42.1
Catering	0	1.1	1.1	1.1
Laundry	0	2.0	0	5.9
Domestic	0.6	3.0	3.0	4.2
Porters	0	8.1	3.2	21.0

Prevalence rates expressed as a percentage of total responses from each category.

Source: Adapted from HSAC 1987, p. 3.

This is such a consistent finding in the literature that surveys differ only by how much more at risk nurses are than other occupational groups. The following studies are typical. Basque and Merhige (1980) surveyed the experiences of 60 nurses working in mental health facilities. Of those questioned, 76 per cent reported that they had encountered verbally abusive and threatening behaviour during the previous week, and 34 per cent reported that they faced such behaviour on a daily basis. Twenty-one per cent of nurses reported that they had weekly contact with residents who were physically aggressive towards them. No details of the grades of staff were given, nor do the authors describe the facilities' or clients' characteristics in any detail. Therefore, we have few clues as to the reasons for this very high rate of aggression.

In a larger study, Rosenthal et al. (1992) surveyed 663 nursing staff in two general hospitals and two hospitals for people with mental health problems. Nurses working in mental health settings had experienced more aggression and violence than their colleagues in general settings. Interestingly, the prevalence of more serious violence was similar in both types of facility. Again, no hypothesis was put forward to suggest why this was the case, and the authors did not compare rates of assault on nurses with those of other professional groups.

Turning to a slightly different setting, Carmel and Hunter (1989) studied reports of injuries to all staff in a hospital for offenders in the United States. Nursing staff were found to have sustained 121 out of the 135 recorded injuries. Finally, in a large-scale survey by the Royal College of Nursing (RCN) (1994) of 1153 community nurses, 336 reported an aggressive incident during the previous year. Only one nurse reported a major incident, and 271 reported incidents of verbal abuse. The study showed that community mental health nurses and health visitors reported encountering the greatest amount of aggression.

The study poses interesting questions about levels of violence in community settings, particularly in the context of discussion over the merits of hospital versus community care. The suggestion from the RCN study is that the level of violence towards community nurses is lower than that towards hospital-based staff. If this is true, it is occurring at a time of significant change in the delivery of health care. In the United Kingdom, the NHS and Community Care Act 1990 (Department of Health 1990) has placed the emphasis on care in community settings, particularly for client groups such as people with learning disability or mental health problems, and older people. Coincidentally, these are the groups that the HSAC survey suggest present the greatest risks to nurses. It could be hypothesised that the move to community settings for these client groups has, by itself, reduced levels of violence. An alternative view is that similar levels of violence exist but that the targets of the violence have changed, perhaps to relatives, the public or other carers. Recent years have witnessed regrettable incidents in which former mental health patients have committed homicide (Boyd 1996), thus raising public fears about the policy of community care. These are complex issues, and our knowledge is incomplete. However, further research is bound to have significant implications for education and policy in this area.

Social workers

Another group of staff who have received attention from researchers are social workers. Like nurses, these staff work in a range of residential and community settings and with different client groups. In early studies, Millham et al. (1976) consulted 394 reports of aggressive incidents in four community homes for boys run by Social Services. The majority of the violence reported was between the residents, and few attacks on staff were uncovered. Breakwell and Rowett (1989) cite a further study by Leavey in 1978, who found that one-third of assaults within 13 children's homes in London were committed against staff. In 1981, the National and Local Government Officers' Association (NALGO) (1983), whose members include social workers, surveyed their branches in the United Kingdom. Of the 221 responses received, only half reported aggression towards them from clients. We do not know what proportion of the incidents involved social workers.

Two studies of violence to social workers deserve special mention. A survey by Brown et al. (1986) of 560 social work staff in 1979 revealed 98 staff who reported at least one attack over the previous 3 years. Also, 134 had been threatened at least once. These figures suggest a lower level of risk compared with that of nurses. However, a study by Rowett (1986) employed a more complex research design in order to estimate the difference between actual and recorded incidents of violence. Rowett first sought information from Social Services departments in the United Kingdom on the number of recorded assaults on social workers. The response rate of 31 per cent showed the prevalence of physical aggression to be one episode for every 259 members of staff. In a follow-up, Rowett then sent questionnaires to 728 social workers in one area. Of the 450 staff who replied, 112 reported that they had been victims of assault. This is at considerable variance to the officially recorded incidence of violence.

Other health workers

Research into aggression towards other professional groups has been less frequent than for nurses and social workers. However, recent well-publicised cases of assaults on general practitioners have renewed interest in this area. As far as the HSAC survey is concerned, general practitioners were the group least at risk of suffering major or minor incidents. A survey of 2684 general practitioners by Hobbs (1991) revealed that, of the 1093 who responded, 63 per cent had been the victim of some sort of aggressive incident during the previous year. Three per cent of respondents had experienced regular minor assaults, and 0.4 per cent had suffered more serious injury. Whereas the prevalence of more serious injury was similar to that revealed by the HSAC survey, Hobbs' study showed that a higher proportion of general practitioners had experienced aggression. However, this has to be seen in the light of a relatively low response to the questionnaire. Nevertheless, the study raises further questions. For example, could the apparent increase in the number of general practitioners at risk be a result of the increasing demands and expectations of the public often claimed to be a consequence of the recent health service reforms?

The figures shown in the HSAC survey for ambulance staff are comparable to those for nursing staff, but there are too few studies in this area to show that this is a consistent finding. Similarly, it is open to speculation why ambulance staff should be a major target of assault. One hypothesis is that ambulance staff are often the first to attend incidents that may have involved violence between members of the public. High levels of arousal among people present at these incidents could easily spill over at the intervention of the ambulance crew. Another factor may be that relatives and friends are often present when staff arrive to attend to a sick or injured person. Their own anxiety and concern could increase the likelihood of aggression. Also, along with social workers, ambulance staff can be involved in the transfer to hospital of people detained under the Mental Health Act. This is often a situation that arouses anger among the people being detained as well as their relatives.

More recent speculation on this issue proposes that the public, particularly younger people, have less respect for authority. Proponents of this view cite examples of attacks on firefighters as well as ambulance staff as evidence for this apparently growing lawlessness. This remains to be proved.

Summary

This section has shown which of the main professional groups of staff are at risk of assault and has concluded that:

- Nursing staff face higher levels of violence than other staff groups
- Nurses working in the community face less violence than their colleagues in hospital or residential services
- Ambulance staff are the group of health service staff facing the second highest levels of violence
- Social workers face higher levels of violence than nurses working in the community.

Client factors

A major suggestion arising out of the HSAC survey is that staff working with people with learning disability and people with mental health problems face the greatest risk of major as well as minor assaults. Does this mean that people with learning disability or mental health problems, by themselves, present greater risks to staff?

People with learning disability

People with learning disability make up approximately 2 per cent of the population. Studies show that a significant group of people with learning disability can display many behaviours that present challenges to staff. This behaviour includes self-injury, damage to property, repetitive or stereotyped behaviour and severe withdrawn behaviour as well as aggression.

Estimates of precisely how many people display challenging behaviour vary considerably. A survey by Jacobsen (1982) puts the figure as high as 73 per cent of all people with learning disability. Other studies (for example, Nihira and Nihira 1975) put the proportion at as low as 16 per cent.

Studies that have looked specifically at violence and aggression are rare and show similar variation. Eyman and Call (1977) found rates of physical aggression as high as 28 per cent of their sample. A more recent survey by Harris (1993) in the south west region of England found prevalence rates of 17.6 per cent for adults and 12.6 per cent for children.

These variations can be accounted for by several factors. Some studies do not successfully differentiate between violence to other people with learning disability and violence to staff or parents. Many people with learning disability will also display more than one type of challenging behaviour, which makes it difficult for researchers to isolate purely aggressive behaviour (Jones and Earys 1993). We also lack qualitative information on the nature of violence perpetrated by people with learning disability. For example, does it differ from that of other people in terms of the intent or hostility displayed at the time? If it does, should it make a difference to the way in which we manage violence? Research on the causes of challenging behaviour suggest that the following factors can increase the likelihood of someone's behaviour being labelled as challenging:

- Staff tolerance and understanding of learning disability
- Understimulating environments
- A poor quality and quantity of interaction with people with learning disability
- Physical causes such as illness or pain that the person cannot communicate.

This list is by no means exhaustive. It supports the view that challenging behaviour is not a static concept but can vary according to the perceptions of staff and the environments in which people find themselves (Hastings *et al.* 1995). Taking this into account, the emphasis in the literature over the previous 10 years on reducing levels of challenging behaviour has stressed the importance of looking for the meaning or function of the person's behaviour (Durand and Crimmins 1991). For example, a person who has no speech may use physical means to get attention. Similarly, a person who is finding a task too difficult may push someone away or throw objects in order to escape the situation.

Anecdotal evidence from studies by MacDonnell *et al.*, cited in MacDonnell and Sturmey (1993, p. 149), also suggests that physical attacks by many people with learning disability are different from the popular image of 'the hardened streetfighter'. All this suggests that we need to consider situations, settings and relationships in looking at the potential for violence.

To summarise, the great variation in estimates of challenging behaviour make it difficult to conclude that people with learning disability, by themselves, consistute a risk to staff. It would be more accurate to point to situational or interpersonal factors to explain the greater prevalence of assault among this group in the HSAC survey. These factors will be explored later in this chapter.

People with mental health needs

In the same way that the HSAC survey raised questions about people with learning disability, people with mental health problems also seem to present significant risks to staff. To what extent is this true?

The public's view of people with mental health problems has been coloured by several heavily publicised cases in recent years of people with a psychiatric diagnosis committing homicide. The atmosphere created by this publicity has been described as one of 'moral panic' (McRobbie and Thornton 1995) in which the whole of the government's policy of community care has been called into question. Some people have tried to put this evidence into perspective by pointing out, for example, that research shows that people with mental health problems are more likely to commit suicide than homicide (Boyd 1996). However, should we need to take steps to minimise risk among certain people with mental health problems?

Researchers looking for possible connections between mental health and violence have tended to focus their attention on people with a diagnosis of schizophrenia. Yesavage (1983) and Tardiff and Sweillam (1980), for example, found that assaults against staff are more likely to be committed by people in an active state of psychosis. Aiken (1984), in his study of 11 violent incidents in a hospital, discovered that delusional beliefs were more likely to be implicated in eight of them. Lion *et al.* (1981), in their study of incidents in a hospital, found that 66 per cent of subjects had a diagnosis of schizophrenia. A report on offenders with a psychiatric diagnosis (Hafner and Boker 1982) also revealed that people with schizophrenia were twice as likely to offend as were other groups of people with mental health problems.

Evidence such as this seems to lend weight to the popular belief that people with schizophrenia are dangerous. However, these studies have simply looked at what proportion of incidents have involved people with schizophrenia. We need to think more broadly about the issue because, as Haller and Deluty (1988) point out:

> discovering that most of the assaultive patients in a particular sample are diagnosed schizophrenic is of little value if most of the *non-assaultive* patients in the sample are also diagnosed schizophrenic. (our italics)

Craig's (1982) study of 172 patients with mental health problems concluded that most people with mental health problems do not commit crimes. However, he also discovered a higher prevalence of offending among people with a history of schizophrenia. Similar findings can be seen in work by Zitrin *et al.* (1976) and Volavka *et al.* (1995). Conclusions reached in these studies suggest that people with schizophrenia who offend have more in common with other people who offend than with other people with schizophrenia. Craig (1982) points to possible social factors that lead people with schizophrenia to offend.

Therefore, the relationship between schizophrenia and violence is more complex than some studies suggest. It is not sufficient to say that this group of people present a greater risk simply because they have such a diagnosis. It is better to say that people with schizophrenia are more likely to be influenced by factors that provoke violence in other people.

Summary

Client factors are not sufficient, in themselves, to explain the risks of violence faced by staff. We need to look more closely at situational or interpersonal factors to understand more clearly why staff are at risk. Since many of the studies of violence to staff have taken place in residential settings, it may be worthwhile looking at factors common to these facilities.

Situational factors

Hospital facilities

Whereas staff can be assaulted in any setting, hospitals present particular security problems (Rogers *et al.* 1999). For example, hospitals often have several entrances and are open 24 hours a day to the public. Many people receiving care in hospital, and sometimes their relatives, may experience stress and thus feel vulnerable, raising the likelihood of aggression. Staff working in some parts of hospitals, such as accident and emergency units, will be at particular risk of assault and abuse. Some of the reasons for this are discussed in Chapter 3. However, accident and emergency departments typically see patients who are in pain and anxious, or disorientated or disinhibited through the influence of drugs or alcohol. These problems can be exacerbated by the length of time it takes before people are treated. Waiting is a well-known cause of frustration, and people are more likely to express this in terms of aggression (Cembrowicz and Shepherd 1992), particularly if they want to show off to their peers.

Residential facilities

We saw above that long-stay residential facilities such as hospitals for people with learning disabilities or mental health problems present greater risks to staff than working in community settings. Rowett's (1986) research into social workers uncovered a similar pattern between field and residential social work and violence, irrespective of the client group being supported. One reason for this, of course, could be that people who are more likely to behave violently are more likely to find themselves in residential facilities. However, research indicates that this may be too simplistic a view: many residential facilities can bring about improvements in quality of life for people whose behaviour presents problems (Emerson and Hatton 1994). On the other hand, we have seen that staff in community settings can face significant levels of violence. Evidence nevertheless shows that residential facilities bring with them risks that can have negative effects on both clients and staff.

As long ago as 1961, Goffman (1961) identified key problems associated with many residential facilities that he called 'total institutions'. These problems are thought to apply mainly to long-stay hospitals and prisons, and will have negative effects upon staff as well as client behaviour. Goffman's ideas have subsequently been supported by other research (King *et al.* 1971) as well as government inquiries into hospitals (see Martin 1984). These problems, or risk factors, can be summarised as follows:

Effects on clients

- A routinised approach to care, allowing little or no choice over daily activities such as what to eat or when to go to bed
- Control of the client's affairs, for example over financial matters, being transferred to the institution
- Restrictions of personal freedom, such as the locking of doors
- Loss of privacy, for example shared bathing areas and large dormitories
- Geographical isolation from communities, thus immunising the institution from the influence of societal norms. For example, contact between the sexes is discouraged
- A routinised approach to care, leading to disorientation in time.

Effects on staff

- Bureaucratic decision-making styles, leaving little room for staff to make changes and respond to clients' wishes
- The disempowerment of staff, who are then unable to empower clients or act as advocates on their behalf
- Remote management decision-making, thus making the process of change very slow
- A 'task'-orientated regimen of care leading to exceptionally low levels of positive interaction between staff and clients
- High levels of staff stress and 'burnout' because of low levels of positive feedback on performance.

Against a background in which tomorrow is expected to be very much the same as today, we should not be surprised that frustration and anger can become dominant emotions in many clients and staff. An opposite reaction is also possible, as shown by Seligman (1975), who invented the term 'learned helplessness' to describe the behaviour of clients who feel no longer able to make any impact on their environment.

Despite the good intentions and sometimes heroic efforts of staff (Slama and Bannerman 1983), it seems clear from Goffman's work that residential services are not the optimum environments to encourage positive, supportive relationships between staff and clients. A key question is how residential facilities can create the circumstances in which violence will take place.

One way of looking at this issue is put forward by Williams (1995), who points out that residential services such as long-stay hospitals reinforce a negative attitude in society that people with learning disability or mental health needs should be segregated from the public. Although many residential facilities are now much smaller and based in community settings, they can still fail to value the people living in them. Simons (1997), for example, points out that, despite the emphasis on homely environments and individualised care, clients can still be regarded as in-patients. Funding sources mean that services are often in the position of both owning the property and having contracts for providing care. Financial incentives mean that services are under pressure to fill places in homes when a client leaves or dies. Therefore, the bed is more important than the person who occupies it. What effects can this have on client and staff relationships, and what is the potential for violence?

In these circumstances, the house in which clients live is not a *home*. There will be little or no choice over whom a client lives with and who works in the house. In this way, residential facilities could be seen as being no different from their larger counterparts described earlier by Goffman. This means that the outcome could be an imbalance of power between staff and clients. We know that staff can feel equally disempowered by the organisations for which they work, which can create risks for clients if staff seek to compensate for their lack of power by exerting inappropriate control over clients (Beardshaw 1981). This is manifested in the physical, sexual, emotional and financial abuse of clients, which has been discussed at length by authors such as Ryan and Thomas (1980) and Hewitt (1987). An equally foreseeable consequence is that clients may challenge the dominance of staff and act out their frustration and anger.

Violent and aggressive responses are not an inevitable consequence of living or working in residential facilities. However, although alternative models of residential support are suggested by Simons (1997) and Kinsella (1993) to redress the imbalance of power, residential facilities will continue to carry the greatest risks.

Professionalism – care or control?

Residential services, then, can teach us a great deal about the nature of relationships between professional staff and clients, and the potential for violence. Other authors have posed more searching questions about the nature of professional practice as a whole. Norris (1990), for example, observes that professionals are increasingly being asked to act in controlling ways on behalf of government. There are more explicit ways in which we can see this taking place. Nurses, psychiatrists and approved social workers have the power to detain people under sections of the Mental Health Act 1983 (Department of Health and Social Security 1983). Social workers also have the power to remove children from families where they suspect the child to be at risk. As far as reactions to this power are concerned, Brown et al. (1986) noted in their research that the majority of violent attacks on social workers happened when they were removing children from parents or escorting people to hospital under a section of the Mental Health Act.

Norris also sees power being exerted over the public by professionals in more subtle ways. He notes that the NHS and Community Care Act 1990 (Department of Health 1990) gave many professionals a role as care manager, with responsibility for assessing needs and allocating resources accordingly. This, argue Norris (1990) and Breakwell (1989), is a gatekeeping role that is incompatible with the role of a professional helper and advocate. No research exists explicitly to link this change in the role of professionals with assaults on them. However, it is not inconceivable that a refusal of a service could generate anger among some clients.

On this issue, Chappell (1992) makes the more general point that it is in the interest of professionals that people continue to use their services. Therefore, creating dependency among clients such as disabled people can help to fulfil the need of professionals to feel wanted and valued. Again, if this perception is an accurate one, we can only surmise that the imbalance of power that this creates could lead to an aggressive response.

Other sources of discontent with professional practice have been noted by Satyamurti (1981). Satyamurti notes that receiving help from someone like a social worker can, in itself, be seen as stigmatising. A great deal of this could be attributed to public stereotypes of professionals such as social workers. Paradoxically, this can result in the client feeling devalued rather than helped and empowered. We certainly need to challenge inaccurate portrayals of professional activity. However, any more additions to the mounting cases of professional failure reported in recent years will make it difficult to instil confidence in professionals once more.

To summarise, it is crucial that professionals use their power responsibly and rediscover a role in which they act in partnership with clients. Residential settings present greater challenges to staff in achieving this, and managers need to be particularly aware of the need to create systems in which staff feel as valued as they hope the service users are. Finally, as Sines (1994) points out, professionals may be unable to resist greater legal responsibilities or a gate-keeping role. However, they should learn not to rely upon formal authority alone when interacting with clients.

Personal factors

So far, we have looked at the occupational, client and situational factors that are thought to create risks of violence for staff. In this final section, we will explore some of the personal characteristics of staff that could expose them to violence.

A question of experience?

As we saw in Table 2.2 above, the amount of violence suffered varied among different grades of staff as well as different types of staff. Student nurses and charge nurses suffered the same levels of major assault, while student nurses were also more likely than other grades of nursing staff to be victims of minor assault and threats. Staff nurses suffered from higher levels of minor injury and threats than did charge nurses. What could account for these differences?

As far as student nurses are concerned, it could be supposed that their inexperience might explain their vulnerability. In a study by Bernstein (1981), inexperienced staff were shown to be assaulted more often than their more senior colleagues. However, a study by Carmel and Hunter (1989) showed that staff who were the most recent employees of the service were the ones more prone to be assaulted. Some of these employees had previous experience in other organisations, suggesting that a knowledge of the clients being cared for could be the major factor in preventing violence. For similar reasons, it might also be supposed that relationships with colleagues and teamworking are also important.

Research has failed to come up with an explanation for why charge nurses might be the grade of nurse as much at risk as their inexperienced student colleagues. It could be the case that those in charge of a ward or area will be more likely to be the first to come to the assistance of colleagues when an incident is taking place. Another explanation is that the person in charge of a facility has the greatest level of formal authority. We have already seen how displays of power over clients can provoke angry responses. The charge nurse may be the person, for example, who more often gives bad news or has to turn down requests from clients.

The position of staff nurse being least at risk is not confirmed by other studies (Lanza 1983, Whittington and Wykes 1994). However, if the HSAC survey is representative, it could be that staff nurses are the group of staff who combine significant levels of personal knowledge of clients with less authority than charge nurses. This may enable them to be better at preventing potential incidents or better at avoiding them. Further research in this area is necessary.

Personal beliefs of staff

Psychological theory and practice have demonstrated that people are not passive observers of events, nor do they simply react to incidents in the environment. Instead, research has shown that all of us hold personal beliefs about the world, which we use to understand what has happened in the past as well as to predict future events (see Marshall and Turnbull 1996). Some attention has been paid to this in research on violence in the workplace.

Rowett (1986), for example, questioned social workers on their beliefs about the characteristics of staff who were most likely to be assaulted at work. He discovered that a commonly held belief was that people who were more prone to assault were authoritarian, inexperienced and overbearing. Interestingly, respondents did not rate *themselves* as having these characteristics, even though they reported that they had been victims of assault. Objective evidence would suggest that anyone can become a victim of violence. However, we know from psychological research that people often ignore evidence when making decisions about their own lives. The implication of this is that it is important for staff to be made aware that anyone can be at risk and thus take necessary precautions.

Davies (1988) has also identified unhelpful beliefs among staff that could have more serious consequences during an incident.

Beliefs about potentially violent clients such as 'If you give them an inch, they'll take a mile' or 'They mustn't be allowed to get away with anything' are probably more common than we would like to admit and are clearly confrontational. It is quite easy to see how beliefs such as these could provoke aggressive responses in themselves as well as others.

A different, but equally unhelpful set of beliefs is also identified by Davies. Some staff will see the need to cope at all costs and hold beliefs such as 'I must never show fear' or 'I must never run away.' Once again, such beliefs could lead to situations in which the member of staff feels obliged to take unacceptable risks.

Gender

Several studies have examined the potential part that the gender of the victim plays in violent attacks. Rowett's (1986) study of social workers showed that male staff were over-represented in reported incidents. Similarly, Carmel and Hunter's (1989) research into violent incidents showed that male staff were twice as likely to suffer assaults as were their female colleagues. One theory for why males are more susceptible is derived from a popular assumption that 'a show of force' towards an aggressor is more likely to bring an incident to an end. Certainly, in hospital settings, males were often called upon to intervene in large numbers when incidents occurred. In some areas, this view may still be held and may increase the risks to male staff. Another reason for the apparent gender imbalance is the conflicting view held by others that women are more successful at de-escalating potentially violent incidents. It is not uncommon, for example, to see greater numbers of women employed by pubs and night clubs.

This view is linked to another commonly held belief that men, although more likely to be the perpetrators of violence, are socialised not to assault women. This belief is not substantiated by research. Whittington and Wykes (1994), in a study in a mental health hospital, discovered that women were just as likely as men to be attacked by male clients in a hospital for people with mental health problems. Furthermore, in their studies of husband's aggression towards their wives, Dobash and Dobash (1979) concluded that the principal motivator in male-to-female aggression seemed to be that men perceived their wives as having failed to live up to their unrealistic expectations. Norris (1990) also suggests that females who are perceived to have power, such as social workers, may represent a threat to men and could be vulnerable to assault.

A similar picture is not replicated as far as women are concerned. Whittington and Wykes' (1994) study discovered that female clients were more likely to attack female than male staff. What is also interesting is that all of the student nurses in the study who were assaulted were the victims of female violence. If the studies above are representative, it would suggest that, whereas men may not discriminate as far as victims are concerned, this is not the case for women. The precise reason for this should be the focus of further research as it could have important implications for the way in which violence is managed.

Personal competence

It could be assumed that staff who have received training and education in the management of violence should be more skilled in managing incidents when they occur. Are we right to make this assumption? Many of the studies into violence towards staff have posed questions about the level of training they have received. The response consistently shows that few have been formally trained. Out of 67 nurses questioned, Basque and Merhige (1980) discovered that three-quarters had received no training in managing aggression. More recently, of the 1153 nurses responding to the RCN survey on violence to community staff (Royal College of Nursing 1994), only a quarter reported that they had been trained in recognising potentially violent incidents or in how to manage them.

However, if violence is a problem, is training the answer? Despite the risks faced by staff, research into the effects of training is rare. Infantino and Musingo (1985) showed that staff in a hospital for people with mental health problems who had undergone training were less likely to suffer assaults than those who had received no training. After only a 2-day training programme, Gertz (1980) discovered that the number of aggressive incidents in a mental health facility fell from 174 to 117. Anecdotal evidence following a 2-week training programme described by Paterson *et al.* (1992) suggested that the increased confidence levels reported by staff contributed to a reduction in the number of incidents.

Although there is some evidence in favour of training, it may not be sufficient, in itself, to reduce the frequency of incidents. A total organisational response may prove to be more effective. This will be taken up in Chapter 10, on the role of the manager.

Conclusion

There is a growing number of research studies that give us valuable insights into the risk factors faced by staff in health and social services. The research shows that nurses in residential settings and social workers in the community face significant risks. This risk is magnified if staff find themselves working with people with learning disabilities who display challenging behaviour, or people with mental health problems. However, we need to bear in mind that the statistics on violence towards staff are a gross underestimate of the actual rate of assault.

We also need to remember that these facts may not give us the whole picture of risk factors. Reflecting on the wealth of research, there is a strong suggestion that factors that have a negative influence on staff/client relationships are more valid predictors of violence than occupational group, client group or setting alone. Although professionals are under ever greater pressure to behave as gatekeepers to services, it should be considered that, if professionals rely upon the exercise of formal authority *alone*, violence will continue to be one of the consequences.

References

Aiken G.J.M. (1984) Assaults on staff in a locked ward: prediction and consequences, *Medicine, Science and the Law*, **24**(3): 199–207.

Basque L.O. and Merhige J. (1980) Nurses' experiences with dangerous behaviour: implications for training, *Journal of Continuing Education in Nursing*, **11**(9): 47–51.

Beardshaw V. (1981) *Conscientious Objectors at Work: Mental Hospital Workers – a Case Study*, London, Social Audit.

Bernstein H.A. (1981) Survey of threats and assaults directed towards psychotherapists, *American Journal of Psychotherapy*, **35**: 243–5.

Boyd W. (1996) *Report of the Confidential Inquiry into Homicides and Suicides by Mentally Ill People*, London, Royal College of Psychiatrists.

Breakwell G. (1989) *Facing Physical Violence*, London, Routledge.

Breakwell G. and Rowett C. (1989) Violence and social work. In Archer J. and Browne K. (eds) *Human Aggression: Naturalistic Approaches*, London, Routledge.

Brown R., Bute S. and Ford P. (1986) *Social Workers at Risk: The Prevention and Management of Violence*, Basingstoke, Macmillan.

Carmel H. and Hunter M. (1989) Staff injuries from inpatient violence, *Hospital and Community Psychiatry*, **40**(1): 41–6.

Castledine G. (1993) Violent attacks: nurses at risk, *British Journal of Nursing*, **2**(3): 187–8.

Cembrowicz S.P. and Shepherd J.P. (1992) Violence in the accident and emergency department, *Medicine, Science and the Law*, **32**: 118–22.

Chappell A.L. (1992) Towards a sociological critique of the normalisation principle, *Disability, Handicap and Society*, **7**(1): 35–54.

Craig T.J. (1982) An epidemiological study of problems associated with violence among pscyhiatric inpatients, *American Journal of Psychiatry*, **139**: 1262–6.

Davies W. (1988) How not to get hit, *Psychologist*, May: 175–6.

Department of Health (1990) *National Health Service and Community Care Act*, London, DoH.

Department of Health and Social Security (1983) *Mental Health Act*, London, HMSO.

Dobash E.R. and Dobash R. (1979) *Women, Violence and Social Change*, London, Routledge.

Durand V.M. and Crimmins D.B. (1991) Teaching functionally equivalent responses as an intervention for challenging behaviour. In Remmington B. (ed.) *The Challenge of Severe Mental Handicap: A Behaviour Analytic Approach*, Chichester, John Wiley & Sons.

Emerson E. and Hatton C. (1994) *Moving Out*, London, HMSO.

Eyman R. and Call T. (1977) Maladaptive behaviour and community placement of mentally retarded persons, *American Journal of Mental Deficiency*, **82**: 137–44.

Gertz B. (1980) Training for prevention of assaultive behaviour in a psychiatric setting, *Hospital and Community Psychiatry*, **31**: 628–30.

Goffman E. (1961) *Asylums: Essays on the Social Situation of Mental Patients and Other Inmates*, New York, Doubleday.

Hafner H. and Boker W. (1982) *Crimes of Violence by Mentally Abnormal Offenders*, Cambridge, Cambridge University Press.

Haller R.M. and Deluty R.H. (1988) Assaults on staff by psychiatric inpatients, *British Journal of Psychiatry*, **152**: 174–9.

Harris P. (1993) The nature and extent of aggressive behaviour amongst people with learning difficulties (mental handicap) in a single health district, *Journal of Intellectual Disability Research*, **37**: 221–42.

Hastings R.P., Remmington B. and Hopper G.M. (1995) Experienced and inexperienced health care workers' beliefs about challenging behaviours, *Journal of Intellectual Disability Research*, **39**(6): 474–83.

Health Services Advisory Committee (1987) *Violence to Staff in the Health Services*, London, HMSO.

Hewitt S. (1987) The abuse of deinstitutionalised persons with mental handicaps, *Disability, Handicap and Society*, **2**: 127–35.

Hobbs F.D.R. (1991) Violence in general practice: a survey of general practitioners' views, *British Medical Journal*, **302**: 329–32.

Infantino J. and Musingo S.Y. (1985) Assaults and injuries among staff with and without training in aggression control techniques, *Journal of Hospital and Community Psychiatry*, **32**: 497–8.

Jacobsen J.W. (1982) Problem behaviour and psychiatric impairment within a developmentally disabled population, 1: behaviour frequency, *Applied Research in Mental Retardation*, **3**: 121–39.

Jones R.S.P. and Earys C.B. (1993) Challenging behaviour and intellectual disability: an overview. In Jones R.S.P. and Earys C.B. (eds) *Challenging Behaviour and Intellectual Disability: A Psychological Perspective*, Clevedon, BILD.

King R.D., Raynes N.V. and Tizard J. (1971) *Patterns of Residential Care: Sociological Studies in Institutions for Handicapped Children*, London, Routledge & Kegan Paul.

Kinsella P. (1993) *Group Homes: An Ordinary Life?* Manchester, National Development Team.

Lanza M.L. (1983) The reactions of nursing staff to physical assault by a patient, *Hospital and Community Psychiatry*, **34**(1): 44–7.

Lion J.R., Snyder W. and Merrill G.L. (1981) Underreporting of assaults on staff in a state hopsital, *Hospital and Community Psychiatry*, **32**: 497–8.

Lipscombe J.A. and Love C.C. (1992) Violence to health care workers: an emerging problem, *American Association of Occupational Health Nursing*, **40**(5): 219–28.

MacDonnell A. and Sturmey P. (1993) Managing violent and aggressive behaviour: towards better practice. In Jones R.S.P. and Earys C.B. (eds) *Challenging Behaviour and Intellectual Disability: A Psychological Perspective*, Clevedon, BILD.

McRobbie A. and Thornton T. (1995) Rethinking moral panic for multi-mediated social worlds, *British Journal of Sociology*, **46**(4): 559–74.

Marshall S. and Turnbull J. (eds) (1996) *Cognitive Behaviour Therapy: An Introduction to Theory and Practice*, London, Baillière Tindall.

Martin J.P. (1984) *Hospitals in Trouble*, Oxford, Blackwell Scientific.

Millham S., Bullock R. and Hosic K.M. (1976) On violence in community houses. In Tutt N. (ed.) *Violence*, London, HMSO.

National and Local Government Officers Association (1983) *Survey and Report on Violence to Members*, London, NALGO.

Nihira L. and Nihira K. (1975) Jeopardy in community placement, *American Journal of Mental Deficiency*, **79**: 538–44.

Norris D. (1990) *Violence Against Social Workers. The Implications for Practice*, London, Jessica Kingsley.

Paterson B., Turnbull J. and Aitken I. (1992) Evaluation of a short course in the management of violence, *Nurse Education Today* **12**: 368–75.

Rogers R., Salvage J. and Cowell R. (1999) *Violence in the Workplace: Nurses at Risk*, 2nd edn, Basingstoke, Macmillan.

Rosenthal T.L., Edwards N.B., Rosenthal R.H. and Ackerman B.J. (1992) Hospital violence: site, severity and nurse's preventative training, *Issues in Mental Health Nursing*, **13**(4): 349–56.

Rowett C. (1986) *Violence in Social Work: A Research Study of Violence in the Context of Local Authority Social Work*, Occasional Paper No. 14, Cambridge, University of Cambridge Institute of Criminology.

Royal College of Nursing (1994) *Violence and Community Nursing Staff*, London, RCN.

Ryan J. and Postner C. (1993) Results of a survey into violence in nursing, *Nursing Times*, **91**(50): 57–61.

Ryan J. and Thomas F. (1980) *The Politics of Mental Handicap*, London, Penguin.

Satyamurti C. (1981) *Occupational Survival*, Oxford, Basil Blackwell.

Seligman M.E.P. (1975) *Helplessness: On Depression, Development and Death*, San Francisco, Freeman.

Simons K. (1997) Residential care or housing and support?, *British Journal of Learning Disabilities*, **25**: 2–6.

Sines D. (1994) The arrogance of power: a reflection on contemporary mental health nursing practice, *Journal of Advanced Nursing*, **20**: 894–903.

Slama K.M. and Bannerman D.J. (1983) Implementing and maintaining a behavioural treatment system in an institutional setting, *Analysis and Intervention in Developmental Disabilities*, **3**: 171–91.

Tardiff K. and Sweillam A. (1980) Assault, suicide and mental illness, *Archives of General Psychiatry*, **37**: 164–9.

Volavka J., Mohammed Y., Vitrai J., Connolly M., Stefanovic M. and Ford M. (1995) Characteristics of state hospital patients arrested for offences committed during hospitalisation, *Psychiatric Services*, **46**(8): 796–800.

Whittington R. and Wykes T. (1994) Violence in psychiatric hospitals: are certain staff prone to being assaulted? *Journal of Advanced Nursing*, **19**: 219–25.

Williams P. (1995) Residential and day services. In Malin N. (ed.) *Services for People with Learning Disabilities*, London, Routledge.

Yesavage J.A. (1983) Bipolar illness: correlates of dangerous inpatient behaviour, *British Journal of Psychiatry*, **143**: 554–7.

Zitrin A., Hardesty A.S. and Burdock E.V. (1976) Crime and violence among mental patients, *American Journal of Psychiatry*, **133**: 142–9.

3

THEORETICAL APPROACHES TO VIOLENCE AND AGGRESSION

John Turnbull

Introduction

The previous chapter discussed the circumstances in which staff are more likely to become victims of violence. This chapter follows on by discussing the circumstances in which people are more likely to become aggressors.

Violence is such a frequent occurrence that it seems a natural part of human behaviour. As such, it occupies a substantial proportion of media attention. The popular view put forward of the causes of violence is that aggressors act out of either 'badness' or 'madness'. For example, we talk of 'mindless' violence, and our sentencing policy towards aggressors reflects a view that people make a conscious decision to inflict harm on others. The key question for us is whether this is a justifiable viewpoint.

For those who are responsible for organising appropriate responses to violence, there is a need to be more objective and to consider the evidence before taking decisions. Therefore, this chapter will discuss the main theoretical approaches to violence and aggression. There have been many perspectives put forward on this subject. Sociologists have looked at the broader issues of violence in society and have sought to influence the development of policies in areas such as crime and sentencing. However, with the exception of the first section on biological influences, the focus in this chapter will be on the key psychological explanations for aggression. These theories tend to give a more individualistic account of the origins of aggressive behaviour, which, we believe, are of more interest to us in developing responses to individuals in our services who behave violently.

A second point to make is that, although some of these theories have achieved greater prominence at certain times in this century, the intention here is not to present them as competing explanations for violence. Instead, you will be invited to consider each one as an influencing factor, capable of interacting with the others to produce a violent or aggressive response.

A biological basis for aggression

The recent advances made in research on genetics have raised the possibility of a greater biological basis for much of human behaviour. It must be said at the outset that the possibility of a biological explanation for social problems such as violence is an attractive one since it implies that individuals could be 'cured' through the use of drugs, surgery or manipulation of genetic material. The reality of the situation, however, is that the research is often conflicting and incomplete. Nevertheless, managers and staff need to be aware of the possibility that physiological changes can account for some episodes of violent behaviour in their services. These will now be discussed in turn.

Neurological factors

Aggression, anger and irritability are well-known consequences of brain injury (Ponsford 1996). Reasons for this are complex and not fully understood. One explanation is that the loss of function that accompanies any serious health problem can be extremely frustrating for the victim. Another explanation is that there has been an injury to a specific area of the brain responsible for regulating anger or aggressive responses. Researchers pursuing this hypothesis have focused their interest on the parts of the brain that make up what is known as the limbic system. Animal research has already provided evidence that surgery or electrical stimulation in this part of the brain can modify aggressive responses. Is this the same for humans?

For ethical reasons, experiments on humans in this area have had to be strictly controlled. Therefore, researchers have tended to focus on individuals with known neurological conditions such as epilepsy or who have suffered some sort of brain trauma such as a tumour. Mark and Irvine (1970) reported on an individual who became violent during complex partial seizures (previously called temporal lobe epilepsy). Electrodes implanted in his brain revealed that this behaviour coincided with discharges in an area of the brain called the amygdala. Similarly, Hitchcock and Cairns (1973) showed that electrical stimulation of the amygdala could arouse rage and escape responses from people. Mark *et al.* (1975) also reported on six patients who had received lesions to the amygdala. For three people, anger and aggressive behaviour ceased, and one person showed a reduction in aggressive behaviour. This evidence seems to lend some support for a possible neurological basis for aggression.

However, other research has not been as encouraging. Balasubraminian *et al.* (1972) studied 128 people who had undergone recent brain surgery. Only nine reported a significant change in their expression of anger. Similarly, Gloor (1972) disputes any association between neurological conditions and violence by pointing out that aggression is not the only response resulting from stimulation of parts of the limbic system. Furthermore, aggression can be the outcome of stimulation of other parts of the brain. This does not totally refute the claim that neurological factors are responsible for some episodes of aggression. It may be that our understanding of precisely how the different parts of the brain interact is incomplete.

A more specific area of research for those seeking a neurological basis for aggression is epilepsy. Gedye (1989), for example, discovered an association between aggression and frontal lobe seizures, although he admits that research is too sparse to draw firm conclusions. The majority of research has focused on complex partial seizures. Early research seemed to show some support for the view that complex partial seizures are responsible for aggressive behaviour. Nuffield (1961) studied 322 children with epilepsy. He found that those with complex partial seizures had the highest incidence of reported aggression. Similarly, Lindsay *et al.* (1979) described a population of 100 people with epilepsy. Thirty-six reported that they had been prone to aggression as children. However, these findings should be treated with caution since some of these people had also suffered brain trauma and some had additional severe mental health problems.

One way of demonstrating a possible link between epilepsy and violence is to study the prevalence of epilepsy among those convicted for violent offences. A survey of offenders by Gunn (1977) showed rates of complex partial seizures to be 7.2 per 1000 of the prison population. This compares with national rates of 9.5 per 1000 (Britten *et al.* 1984). Obviously, this does not support an association between epilepsy and violent offending.

Even though research such as this builds up a picture of a tenuous link between epilepsy and aggression, investigators have not been discouraged. Much of the research has tended to look for an association between violence and epilepsy at the moment when the seizure takes place. When this does occur, the evidence is that the aggression is 'disordered, unco-ordinated and non-directed' (Fenwick 1986, p. 41). Therefore, other researchers have looked for behavioural changes in the interval between seizures. Rodin's (1973) survey of 700 records of people with complex partial seizures showed that only 5 per cent had shown aggression in the period between seizures. Finally, a major international study carried out by Delgado-Escueta *et al.* (1981) sought to come up with the final word on the issue of aggression and epilepsy. In 5400 videotapes of seizures studied, only 13 cases of violence were discovered. Statistically speaking, this is not sufficient to demonstrate a link. In fact, this shows that the prevalence of aggression among people with epilepsy is low.

To conclude this brief discussion, there is little evidence to establish a firm link between neurological conditions and aggression. This does not necessarily mean that, in the future, a link will not be found. One difficulty, as Corsellis (1970) points out, is that brain trauma does not confine itself neatly to the areas of the brain thought to regulate aggression. Furthermore, in their review of the literature, Kligman and Goldberg (1975) are severely critical of the research methods used by investigators. Also facing researchers into epilepsy is the problem that the technology used to record epileptic seizures can be unreliable. It may be that advances in technology will produce more conclusive results.

Hormonal factors

Another argument put forward by those who support a biological basis for aggression is the fact that there appears to be a significant difference in the rate of violence between men and women, a difference that cannot be denied. Official crime statistics (see Home Office 1993) show that men are seven times more likely to commit violent offences than women, and to do so with a greater degree of severity. Even when these figures are compared with surveys of self-reported offending (Farrington 1994), significant differences still exist.

The likelihood of men behaving more aggressively could be explained by the fact that men are generally stronger and taller than women, which may encourage them to behave in more domineering ways. This idea has not been investigated in detail. However, an unexpected finding from Rowett's survey (1986) was that aggressors were usually shorter than their victims.

Some researchers have looked for a possible link between the male hormone, testosterone, and violent behaviour. Kreuz and Rose (1972) investigated young offenders and discovered some association between testosterone levels and aggressive behaviour. Official statistics on violent offending also lend some support to this view. For example, recent evidence suggests that the peak age for conviction for all offences in England and Wales is 18 years for males and 15 years for females. The Cambridge study of delinquent behaviour carried out by Farrington and West (1990) showed that the average age for violent offences among men was 20 years. From biological research, we already know that testosterone levels in the body rise during puberty and reach their peak in the late teens. This is suggestive of a link, although other research shows that this relationship is not as simple as it might appear.

In their studies on monkeys, Rose et al. (1975) discovered that testosterone levels were raised when monkeys had engaged in domineering behaviour over others. Monkeys who became submissive showed reduced levels of testosterone. This finding was replicated in Kedenburg's (1979) study of United States naval officers. He discovered that officers had lower than normal testosterone levels on entry to training. As they progressed through college, these levels rose. This led Kedenburg to the conclusion that testosterone has more to do with dominance than with aggression, although aggression may be one of the strategies used by men to establish their dominance.

Genetic factors

Interest in the possible genetic determinants of aggression heightened in the 1970s following the discovery that men with an extra Y chromosome were over-represented in secure psychiatric hospitals. Since the Y chromosome is the one that determines male characteristics, this could indicate an association between masculinity and aggression. However, further investigations revealed that the presence of an extra chromosome was, if anything, more likely to be associated with property offences than violent crime (Casey et al. 1973). This research also established that, although residents of secure facilities were 30 times more likely to have an extra chromosome, there were also considerable numbers of other people with an extra Y chromosome living perfectly law-abiding lives in society. Therefore, the presence of the extra chromosome is not sufficient, in itself, to make an individual behave violently.

Other physiological changes

Staff working in health and social care settings have often reported an association between aggressive behaviour and the physiological changes brought about by alcohol and drugs: a visit to an accident and emergency department on a Saturday night will bear witness to this. However, what does the research evidence have to say?

Studies by Walker *et al.* (1981) have shown that aggressive responses can be heightened when people are under the influence of drugs such as amphetamines. However, this is not the case for all narcotic substances. Investigations into people who use cannabis, for example, has shown that users often appear to be mild mannered and placid individuals. It could, of course, be possible that people who have more passive or submissive personalities are attracted to this type of drug. However, research by Bailey *et al.* (1983), using a random sample of the population, showed that the use of cannabis can decrease feelings of aggression.

Alcohol is another substance that is known to be implicated in violent offences (Kroll and McKenzie 1983). However, research has yet to establish precisely how alcohol misuse leads to violence. For example, it has been found that expectations play a large part in how we behave under the influence of alcohol. In a well-known study by Powers and Kutash (1978), subjects were divided into two groups, one being told they would be given a drink containing alcohol and the other being told they would be given tonic water. In reality, half of each group was given alcohol and the other half tonic water. Experimenters then set about trying to provoke one of the groups while, in the other, normal conversation was maintained. Interestingly, the people in the group who drank tonic water but thought it was alcohol behaved in a more uninhibited fashion and more aggressively. Levels of provocation were not as significant an influence on behaviour as the expectations held by people about how they should behave under the influence of alcohol.

Setting conditions also have an important role to play in other expressions of violence. For example, if a group of habitually violent football fans drink heavily prior to a football match and find themselves in a fight following the match, what has caused the violence? It could be that being in a large group at a football match and the fact that violence increases their feelings of dominance are the more probable motivators for their violence. The role that alcohol plays in this scenario is one of an accelerant.

Similarly, Raistrick (1994) has shown that between 50 and 90 per cent of violent incidents in domestic settings in North America occur when at least one of the participants is intoxicated. Can we say, however, that alcohol has caused the aggression? It is more likely that alcohol is accelerating the deterioration of an already failing relationship (Gayford 1994).

To summarise this section, biological factors have some links with violent behaviour. However, it unclear precisely how they interact with other factors such as social or psychological influences. It is to those influences which we now turn.

Instinct theories

The early 'instinctivists'

The idea that humans act out of instinct or often seem 'driven' in some aspects of their behaviour was one of the earliest explanations for aggression. This school of thought later became known as instinctivism (Fletcher 1968). One of the earliest exponents of instinctivism was McDougall (1947), who developed what has become known as the hydraulic model of human behaviour (Figure 3.1).

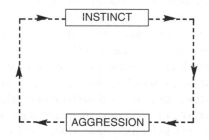

Figure 3.1   Model of instinct theory of aggression

Within this model, it is proposed that humans can be likened to vessels in which the emotions build up to a point at which they must be released. Once purged of this emotion, the pressure can build once more. The idea of a build-up of tension followed by a sudden release has some validity. After all, violent outbursts are often said to occur with no apparent cause, and the intensity of the reaction may seem out of proportion to any provocation. Similarly, we often talk of people 'blowing their top', and we employ strategies such as physical exercise to 'let off steam'.

However elegant these metaphors seem, McDougall and his colleagues' explanation does not answer all of our questions about violence. For example, why are some people more aggressive than others? Is it that habitually violent people experience more stressors than others or that they have fewer outlets to release the built-up tension? How long does it take for someone to build up sufficient tension to want to be violent? Unfortunately, McDougall provides no experimental evidence to support his theory. However, he acknowledged that personal experience might have some effect on developing instinctive responses and that individual factors needed to be accounted for. This is important, since it is then theoretically possible to alter the environment to modify aggressive behaviour.

Sigmund Freud

Although Freud had developed his theories of human behaviour before McDougall, it was later in his career that he turned his attention more specifically to aggression and violence in order to modify the early instinctivist theories.

Like his contemporaries, Freud believed that humans were governed by instincts that he claimed were located in their subconscious mind. Problems in a person's behaviour in adult life were thought to be the outcome of traumatic experiences in childhood. This differs from McDougall's view by placing greater emphasis on individual experiences. From his interaction with his patients, Freud hypothesised that there were two main instincts governing behaviour: the sex and self-preservation instincts. The sex instinct drove people to seek pleasure. However, in the real world, total freedom to satisfy this instinct does not exist. The possibility of behavioural excess is, therefore, curbed by the instinct for self-preservation. Freud labelled this the reality principle. Again, this develops McDougall's ideas by, at least, giving us an explanation why some people seem able to control their instincts better than others.

Freud's theories and interests altered significantly during the 1920s and 30s. He began to give more serious attention to issues such as violence as a direct result, some (Fromm 1977) claim, of experiencing the destructiveness of World War I. His sex and self-preservation instincts were reconceptualised as an instinct for life and death. Aggression and violence, he believed, were under the control of the latter and could be turned inwards by the person, resulting in self-destructive behaviour.

A key question is to what extent Freud's theories help us to understand why one of our patients or clients would turn to violence? As with McDougall's model, the power and spontaneity of some people's reactions adds weight to the notion that violence is governed by internal forces rather than external events. We also know that many of the people whom we help and support have experienced traumatic events earlier in their lives that we believe have affected them significantly. In some ways, it might also be convenient for staff to explain away someone's actions by blaming their instincts or subconscious motivation rather than sharing any responsibility for incidents. In truth, Freud's theories are given little attention by academics and researchers seeking explanations for violence. This is for three main reasons. First, his deterministic theories of human beings offer few opportunities to change an individual's behaviour and, therefore, manage violence more successfully. Second, Freud relied almost entirely on his own subjective experiences of people displaying extreme examples of distress. It is difficult to generalise from these exceptional examples to the whole population. Finally, by today's standards, Freud provided little in the way of objective evidence to prove his theory.

Konrad Lorenz

In spite of some of the difficulties with instinct theory, interest in it has persisted throughout the twentieth century. In fact, one of the most influential publications on aggression was written by Konrad Lorenz (1966), a leading instinctivist. Lorenz's approach to the subject was derived from a discipline known as ethology. Ethologists study the behaviour of animals in the wild and try to discover the function that each behaviour serves for the animal.

Using an ethological framework, Lorenz proposed that humans are naturally aggressive. Although compelled by their instincts to behave aggressively, Lorenz noted that humans could use various outlets for these feelings. Thus, he saw no difference between expressions of physical or verbal aggression. The interesting aspect of Lorenz's theory is that he is practically the only writer not to see aggression in a wholly negative way. For example, he points to competitive sport and competition between businesses as modern-day expressions of a primitive instinct for self-preservation or survival of the fittest. On the other hand, Lorenz pointed out that modern life had created the potential for greater destruction. For example, there is a world of difference between two people fighting over a piece of land and generals committing nuclear missiles to civilian targets in another country. To counteract this destructive potential, Lorenz recommended that any aggressive instincts should be channelled more constructively on both an individual and a societal level. He was a great believer, for example, in global sporting events such as the Olympic Games. He also called on society to reward and encourage the development of what ethologists would call 'appeasement' behaviours. In their study of animals, ethologist noted that conflicts are often avoided when one animal decides to back down at the prospect of a fight. Lorenz believed that this, too, was a natural instinct, which society had failed to encourage in people.

As with other instinctivists, Lorenz's ideas have been seen as extremely credible explanations for violent behaviour. Business can often be conducted in what seems an aggressive atmosphere of 'cut-throat' competition. Furthermore, given our access to the media, we could be forgiven for believing that conflict between groups in society and between nations seems an inevitable part of life. On the other hand, critics have pointed to the fact that Lorenz developed his ideas at a time when the threat of the destruction of the whole planet through nuclear weapons was a very real possibility. This, claim some, took away some of his objectivity. From a theoretical point of view, his fellow ethologists (Siann 1985) have criticised his approach for misrepresenting their discipline. They emphasise the importance of environmental events in developing animal behaviour, accusing Lorenz of focusing too much on instincts.

Drive theories

Frustration

So far, we have seen how those looking for the origins of aggression and violence have focused on the characteristics of the individual aggressor. From a theoretical viewpoint, this approach has some validity. From a moral point of view, this approach has also been popular among those who believe that individuals should be held accountable for their actions. However, other theorists have taken a different approach by looking at the influence of the environment on aggressive behaviour. The remainder of this chapter will be spent discussing these approaches.

One of the first people to consider the effects of the environment on aggressive behaviour was Dollard (Dollard *et al.* 1939). Dollard's central idea was that every incident of aggression was the result of frustration. He believed that all human behaviour was essentially goal directed; this could range from someone simply setting out one morning with the objective of getting to work to the more complex goal of becoming a highly successful manager. Anything that interrupts an objective being attained will be seen as frustrating and is likely to lead to an aggressive response. Dollard's model is explained in Figure 3.2.

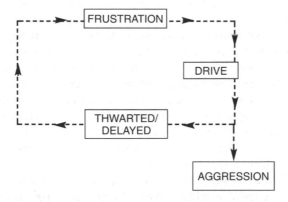

Figure 3.2   Frustration model of aggression

This view of human behaviour has become known as drive theory. Like the instinctivists, the drive theorists believe that all of us have an innate characteristic that compels us to pursue our own goals. However, the theory differs in that the trigger for aggression depends upon factors external to the individual. For example, we are unlikely to behave aggressively if we manage to travel to work on time. However, if an accident occurs that will make us late, this is likely to provoke an angry response. Dollard's explanation for the aggression is simply that environmental factors rather than individuals are responsible for the aggression.

To support this view of aggression, Siann (1985) quotes a number of experiments. In an early study, a group of children were allowed access to a room full of toys while another group of children were delayed access to the toys and had to watch the others playing with them. Observers of the behaviour of the two groups concluded that the second group played in a more aggressive and destructive fashion. Other evidence for the effects of frustration has come from Sheridan *et al.* (1990). These authors showed that a substantial amount of aggression in mental health facilities occurred when staff were seen to enforce the rules of the service. Similarly, Hobbs (1994) demonstrated that being kept waiting, for example to see a doctor, could be a major precipitator of aggressive feelings. In Novaco's (1978) extensive work on anger, frustration was listed as one of the main causes of anger among people.

As with other theories of aggression, staff working in human services will recognise instances when violence has been the result of someone's frustration. However, Dollard's theory also raises questions about its application to all incidents of aggression. In other words, does frustration always lead to aggression? As we saw in Chapter 2, institutional cultures can bring about an opposite reaction in that some individuals will become withdrawn and submissive when requests are turned down. Even if we accept that frustration always leads to aggression, some people seem to be able to tolerate a high degree of frustration while others seem to have a shorter 'fuse'. Dollard failed to account for these individual differences. Another issue is whether we need to be consciously aware of our goals in order for events to be perceived as frustrating. Again, Dollard took little account of this issue.

Some of these issues have been taken up by other researchers, such as Buss (1966), who showed that there is a relationship between frustration and aggression but that it is not always a straightforward one. In one of his experiments, Buss told a group of students that they were going to take part in an experiment to find out how learning could be improved. To do this, each student was paired with another person who sat behind a screen. Unbeknown to the students, the partners chosen for them were members of the team of investigators. The students were told to read out questions for their partner to answer. If their partner got the wrong answer, the students were given a 'dummy' machine through which they could administer an electric shock to see whether this gave their partner extra motivation to answer correctly. One group of students were told that their own psychology grades at the university depended on them doing well on this task. The other group were told nothing. The results showed that the first group were more likely to administer higher degrees of electric shock to their partner. Thus, although both groups were frustrated in completing their task by their partners giving wrong answers to questions, aggressive behaviour is more likely to be a consequence when people are aware of its usefulness in achieving a desired goal.

From experiments like these, Buss went on to question other possible motives for aggression. For example, he asked whether there was a difference between someone who hits out at a person after being provoked and someone who hits out at someone during a robbery. According to Buss, the former example is one of 'angry aggression' and the latter one of 'instrumental aggression'. From a theoretical point of view, this distinction is important and builds on the approaches of other theorists who have looked for a single explanation for aggression. From a practical point of view, it also gives us some insight into how violent and aggressive behaviour might be better managed in services. For example, it could be hypothesised that angry aggression is the type more likely to be encountered by staff. Thus, a major goal of staff would be to reduce levels of provocation. This idea will be taken up in more detail in later chapters of this book. The distinction also helps us identify possible motives in people who are habitually violent and to devise more appropriate long-term strategies. This topic is beyond the scope of this book, but interested readers are referred to discussions by Goldstein and Keller (1987).

Social learning theory

Behaviourism

The significance of Dollard's and Buss's approach lay in moving attention away from personal to environmental factors to explain aggression. Buss's experiments also highlighted the possibility that people could behave aggressively in the anticipation of some sort of reward. Experimental support for this view began with the work of Pavlov (1927) and Watson (1913), who founded a branch of psychology that became known as behaviourism. Pavlov, in a famous experiment, showed how a dog could be made to salivate at the sound of a bell. The dog had previously been given food at the same time as a bell rang. Eventually, the dog could be conditioned to salivate simply at the sound of the bell. Later, B.F. Skinner (1953) developed behaviourism to the point at which it has had a major impact on approaches to many personal and social problems.

Skinner proposed that all behaviour is learned. In order to initiate behaviour, there must first of all be a stimulus, or trigger, in the environment. In terms of aggression, this stimulus might be a receptionist telling us that we will have to wait an hour before seeing a doctor. Responses to stimuli depend on the consequences that have been applied to the behaviour in the past. For example, if we shout at the receptionist and she gives in, letting us see the doctor immediately, we have learned that shouting brings us want we want. In this example, our behaviour has been positively reinforced. On the other hand, if the receptionist tells us that we will have to wait another half an hour, the likelihood of resorting to shouting in the future will decrease. In this instance, our behaviour has been punished. Much of our behaviour, says Skinner, is also maintained through a process of negative reinforcement in which a behaviour is performed to avoid or escape from an aversive situation. For example, a parent might buy sweets for a child in a supermarket queue to avoid a temper tantrum. In terms of aggression, people may also resort to violence to try to bring an end to a situation they find intolerable. In the face of the intimidating behaviour of a bully, some people resort to aggression, not to prove how much tougher they are than the bully, but to seek to bring an end to it or to avoid humiliation. From our discussion of the disempowering nature of human services, this could explain why violence becomes the chosen option for disempowered clients.

The major impact of behaviourism has been that it presents opportunities to change behaviour by altering the antecedents or consequences for behaviour. However, it has also criticised, not least for apparently reducing human behaviour to a series of stimuli and responses. Although behaviourism has amassed considerable support for its principles in the research literature (Iwata *et al.* 1982), problems with applying these principles have been equally highlighted for many years. Salter (1949), for example, reported problems in replicating in humans the early behavioural experiments on animals. However, it was Tolman and Honzik (1930) who showed that the motivation for behaviour might not be as simple as behaviourists first intimated. In one of their experiments, Tolman and Honzik took three groups of rats and observed their behaviour going through a maze. The first group were rewarded with food upon completion of the maze. The second group were given no reinforcement for completing the journey. As the behaviourists would predict, the first group increasingly made fewer errors than the second group. However, the third group of rats were given no reward for their first 10 trips through the maze but were then rewarded for subsequent journeys. It was discovered that this group were able to 'catch up' with the performance of the first group even though they had only been reinforced for half of the journeys. Tolman and Honzik concluded that learning had been taking place in the rats even though they had not been rewarded for it. They hypothesised that the rats might have been constructing a 'mental map' of the maze that enabled them to make fewer errors later on. Therefore, although reinforcement is an important motivator for behaviour, learning can also take place via other means.

Albert Bandura

This view that people's motivation can come from intrinsic as well as extrinsic sources has been taken up by other researchers. Deci (1975), for example, demonstrated that people's performance increased when they were engaged in a task in which they were more interested. However, it was Albert Bandura (1973) who developed these ideas further and gave us a theory that social scientists have found to be more useful in explaining social behaviour such as aggression. His model, called social learning theory, is shown in Figure 3.3.

One of the problems with Skinner's views is that he seemed to suggest that behaviour that has not been directly reinforced or punished cannot be learned. Like Tolman, Bandura showed that learning can take place through a variety of means. This includes learning through our knowledge of what happens to other people. In other words, people can provide us with models of behaviour that we feel motivated to imitate. This knowledge not only may be acquired through directly observing others, but could also come from media images or even by reading about the actions of others.

In a now key experiment (Bandura *et al.* 1963), young children were shown a film of adults behaving aggressively towards a doll. When given a similar doll to play with, it was observed that the children copied the adults' behaviour. Bandura's experiment would seem to lend weight to the current argument that violent images via videos or television could be responsible for the perceived increase in violence in our society. However, an important finding from Bandura's work was that people are more likely to want to copy others' behaviour if they feel that there is an association between themselves and those whom they observe. Another point made by Bandura was that aggression would only be copied in situations where the individual felt aroused and where he or she felt the use of aggression to be justified.

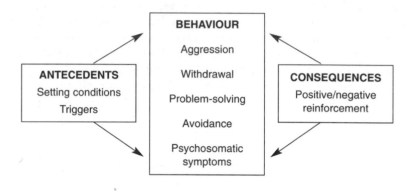

Figure 3.3   Model of social learning theory of aggression

There is some evidence from human service settings to support Bandura's views. Weaver *et al.* (1978) discovered that violence in a mental health facility followed peaks and troughs, and suggested that some residents were copying the behaviour of others. Another explanation for the extent of violence in human services, although not empirically tested, is that the public have learned that assaulting doctors, nurses or social workers brings few punishments or sanctions. For example, assaulting a police officer will bring with it a severe sanction from the courts, but why should the public have a different view of assaults on other public workers such as health service staff?

Cognitive-behavioural approaches

The work of Bandura and Tolman opened up our view of behaviour to consider the role played by internal processes in learning, such as thoughts and beliefs. This work led to the development of a branch of psychological theory known as cognitivism, in which behaviour is thought to be influenced primarily by people's cognitions, for example thoughts, beliefs and expectations. In other words, our behaviour is not governed by events but by the way in which we interpret them. The model in Figure 3.4 shows how the interaction of external events, internal process and emotions combines to produce behaviour.

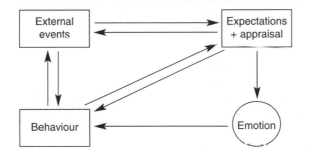

Figure 3.4   Cognitive-behavioural model of aggression

Cognitive theory has contributed immensely to helping people to overcome psychological problems and now has a substantial amount of research to support its use (see Marshall and Turnbull 1996). In terms of aggression and violence, the work of Raymond Novaco (1978) has been highly influential. Using the model in Figure 3.4, Novaco proposed that not all events are intrinsically provoking: it is the way in which events are interpreted that arouses anger and irritation. Much of our behaviour is based on funda-mental beliefs, or constructs, about the world. For example, many of us believe that the world should be a fair place in which to live. However, there are many examples from everyday life in which this belief might be challenged. Most of us prevent ourselves becoming angry at these events by other beliefs such as 'I can't always get what I want' or 'You can't win them all.' Thus, we are able to think flexibly and adjust our expectations. According to Novaco, difficul-ties arise because people are unable to react like this all the time. For example, a nurse who sticks rigidly to the belief that 'Nurses should be able to cope with everything' is running the risk of disappointment and loss of confidence as his or her behaviour cannot possibly live up to these expectations.

Another key feature of the cognitive model is that people are very selective in taking in information (Novaco and Welsh 1989). In other words, people will pay more attention to events that confirm their beliefs than disconfirm them. This explains why some people persist with ways of behaving that appear self-defeating or seem to elicit little or no reinforcement. On the one hand, this can lead to high levels of achievement. On the other, it can be the cause of highly destructive and antagonistic behaviour. Imagine a man who has contacted the Social Services department for help. A social worker has made an assessment of his circumstances and concludes that he is not entitled to the service. If he believes that people just want to put him down all the time, the social worker's decision will be appraised, or interpreted, as a personal attack rather than a professional simply applying the rules. If he holds another belief that unfairness, or wrong-doing, should be punished, he would then see aggression as a justified response. When interviewed about their reasons for hitting out at another person, or even in cases of murder, aggressors have often replied that the victim deserved to be hit (Howells 1989).

As in the case of behaviourism, cognitive theory has been a highly influential and popular approach to understanding human aggression. With its emphasis on the individual, its approach presents a humanistic and optimistic view of people by suggesting that beliefs, and therefore behaviour, can be modified.

Conclusion

It has only been possible here to set out the briefest discussion of the main theoretical approaches to violence and aggression. However, we have seen how theorists have focused on two essential explanations for violent and aggressive behaviour. The first is an approach that looks at internal factors and considers violent behaviour to be caused by innate characteristics such as instinct and drive. The second approach considers the influence of external factors such as the environment and the behaviour of others. No attempt has been made to prove the superiority of one theory over another. Most of these approaches have been well articulated and supported by substantial research. However, the relatively recent development of cognitive explanations for behaviour is interesting in that they appear to provide an explanation that unifies the influences of both external and internal factors. What is clear is that further research is needed to develop our understanding of the origins of aggressive behaviour as well as the development of our own skills in reflecting on our experiences.

References

Bailey D.S., Leonard K.E., Cranston J.W. and Taylor S.P. (1983) Effects of alcohol and self-awareness on human physical aggression, *Personality and Social Psychology Bulletin*, **9**: 289–95.

Balasubraminian V., Ramanujam P.B., Kanaka T.S. and Ramamurthis B. (1972) Stereotaxic surgery for behaviour disorder. In Hitchcock L., Laitinen L. and Vaernet K. (eds) *Psychosurgery*, Springfield, IL, Charles C. Thomas.

Bandura A. (1973) *Aggression: A Social Learning Analysis*, New Jersey, Prentice-Hall.

Bandura A., Ross D. and Ross S.A. (1963) Imitation of film-mediated aggressive models, *Journal of Abnormal and Social Psychology*, **66**: 3–11.

Britten N., Wadsworth M. and Fenwick P. (1984) Stigma in patients with early epilepsy: a national longitudinal study, *Journal of Epidemiology and Community Health*, **38**: 291–5.

Buss A.W. (1966) Instrumentality of aggression, feedback and frustration and determinants of physical aggression, *Journal of Personality and Social Psychology*, **3**: 153–162.

Casey M.D., Black C.E., McLean T.M. *et al.* (1973) Male patients with chromosome abnormality in state hospitals, *Journal of Mental Deficiency Research*, **16**: 215–56.

Corsellis J.A.N. (1970) The pathological anatomy of the temporal lobe with special reference to the limbic areas. In Price J.H. (ed.) *Modern Trends in Psychological Medicine*, No. 2, London, Butterworth.

Deci E.L. (1975) *Intrinsic Motivation*, New York, Plenum Press.

Delgado-Escueta A., Mattson R. and King L. (1981) The nature of aggression during epileptic seizures, *New England Journal of Medicine*, **61**: 333–7.

Dollard J., Doob L.W., Miller N.E., Mowrer O.H. and Seers R.R. (1939) *Frustration and Aggression*, New Haven, Yale University Press.

Farrington D.P. (1994) The cause and prevention of offending, with special reference to violence. In Shepherd J. (ed.) *Violence in Health Care*, Oxford, Oxford University Press.

Farrington D.P. and West D.J. (1990) The Cambridge study in delinquent behaviour. A long term follow-up of 411 London males. In Kerner H.J. and Kaiser G. (eds) *Criminality, Personality, Behaviour and Life History*, Berlin, Springer Verlag.

Fenwick P. (1986) Aggression and epilepsy. In Trimble M.R. and Bolwig T.G. (eds) *Aspects of Epilepsy and Psychiatry*, Chichester, John Wiley & Sons.

Fletcher R. (1968) *Instinct in Man*, London, Allen & Unwin.

Fromm E. (1977) *The Anatomy of Human Destructiveness*, Harmondsworth, Penguin.

Gayford J. (1994) Domestic violence. In Shepherd J. (ed.) *Violence in Health Care*, Oxford, Oxford University Press.

Gedye A. (1989) Episodic rage and aggression attributed to frontal lobe seizures. *Journal of Mental Deficiency Research*, **33**: 369–79.

Gloor P. (1972) Temporal lobe epilepsy: its possible contribution to the understanding of the functional significance of the amygdala and of its interaction with neurocortical temporal mechanisms. In Eletheriou B. (ed.) *The Neurobiology of the Amygdala*, Plenum Press, New York.

Goldstein A.P. and Keller H. (1987) *Aggressive Behaviour: Assessment and Intervention*, London, Pergammon Press.

Gunn J. (1977) *Epileptics in Prison*, London, Academic Press.

Hitchcock E. and Cairns V. (1973) Amygdalotomy, *Postgraduate Medical Journal*, **49**: 894–904.

Hobbs F.D.R. (1994) Aggression towards general practitioners. In Whykes T. (ed.) *Violence and Health Care Professionals*, London, Chapman & Hall.

Home Office (1993) *Criminal Statistics: England and Wales*, London, HMSO.

Howells K. (1989) Anger management methods in relation to the prevention of violent behaviour. In Archer J. and Browne K. (eds) *Human Aggression: Naturalistic Approaches*, London, Routledge.

Iwata B.A., Dorsey M.F., Slifer K.J., Bauman K.E. and Richman G.S. (1982) Towards a functional analysis of self-injury, *Analysis and Intervention in Developmental Disabilities*, **2**: 3–20.

Kedenburg D. (1979) Testosterone and human aggression: an analysis, *Journal of Human Evolution*, **8**: 407–10.

Kligman D. and Goldberg D.A. (1975) Temporal lobe epilepsy and aggression, *Journal of Nervous and Mental Diseases*, **160**: 324–41.

Kreuz L.E. and Rose R.M. (1972) Assessment of aggressive behaviour and plasma testosterone in a young criminal population, *Psychosomatic Medicine*, **34**: 321–2.

Kroll J. and McKenzie T.B. (1983) When psychiatrists are liable: risk management of violent patients, *Hospital and Community Psychiatry*, **34**: 29–36.

Lindsay J., Ounstead C. and Richards P. (1979) Long-term outcome in children with temporal lobe seizures, 3: Psychiatric aspects in childhood and adult life, *Developmental Medicine and Child Neurology*, **21**: 630–6.

Lorenz K. (1966) *On Aggression*, London, Methuen.

McDougall T.W. (1947) *The Energies of Men*, 7th edn, London, Methuen.

Mark V.H. and Ervin F. (1970) *Violence and the Brain*, London, Harper & Row.

Mark V.H., Sweet W. and Ervin F. (1975) Deep temporal lobe stimulation and destructive lesions in episodically violent temporal lobe epileptics. In Fields W. and Sweet W. (eds) *Neural Bases of Violence and Aggression*, St Louis, Warren H. Greem.

Marshall S. and Turnbull J. (eds) (1996) *Cognitive Behaviour Therapy: An Introduction to Theory and Practice*, London, Baillière Tindall.

Novaco R.W. (1978) Anger and coping with stress. In Foreyt J.P. and Rathzen D.P. (eds) *Cognitive Behaviour Therapy*, New York, Plenum Press.

Novaco R.W. and Welsh W.N. (1989) Anger disturbances: cognitive mediation and clinical prescriptions. In Howells K. and Hollin C. (eds) *Clinical Approaches to Violence*, Chichester, John Wiley & Sons.

Nuffield E. (1961) Neurophysiology and behaviour disorders in epileptic children, *Journal of Mental Science*, 107: 438–58.

Pavlov I.P. (1927) *Conditioned Reflexes: An Investigation of the Physiological Activity of the Cerebral Cortex*, New York, Dover.

Ponsford J. (1996) Mechanisms, recovery and sequelae of traumatic brain injury: a foundation for the REAL approach. In Ponsford J. (ed.) *Traumatic Brain Injury. Rehabilitation for Everyday Adaptive Living*, Hove, Psychology Press.

Powers R.J. and Kutash I.L. (1978) Substance-induced aggression. In Kutash I.L. and Kutash L.B. (eds) *Violence: Perspectives on Murder and Aggression*, San Fransisco, Jossey Bass.

Raistrick D. (1994) Alcohol, other drugs and violence. In Shepherd J. (ed.) *Violence in Health Care*, Oxford, Oxford University Press.

Rodin E.A. (1973) Psychomotor epilepsy and aggressive behaviour, *Archives of General Psychiatry*, 28: 210–13.

Rose R.M., Bernstein I.S. and Gordon J.P. (1975) Consequences of social conflict on plasma testosterone levels in rhesus monkeys, *Psychosomatic Medicine*, 47: 173–8.

Rowett C. (1986) *Violence in Social Work*, Occasional Paper No. 14, Cambridge Institute of Criminology, Cambridge, Cambridge University Press.

Salter A. (1949) *Conditioned Reflex Therapy*, New York, Strauss & Young.

Sheridan M., Henrion R., Robinson L. and Baxter V. (1990) Precipitants of violence in a psychiatric inpatient setting. *Hospital and Community Psychiatry*, 41(7): 776–80.

Siann G. (1985) *Accounting for Aggression*, London, Allen & Unwin.

Skinner B.F. (1953) *Science and Human Behaviour*, New York, Free Press.

Tolman E.C. and Honzik C.H. (1930) Introduction and removal of a reward and maze learning in rats, *Psychology*, 4: 257–75.

Walker S., Yesavage A. and Tinklenberg J.R. (1981) Acute phencyclidine (PCP) intoxication: quantitative urine levels and clinical management, *American Journal of Psychiatry*, 138: 674–5.

Watson J.B. (1913) Psychology as a behaviourist views it, *Psychological Review*, 20: 158–77.

Weaver S.M., Broome A.K. and Kat B.J.B. (1978) Some patterns of disturbed behaviour in a closed ward environment, *Journal of Advanced Nursing*, 3: 251–63.

4

LEGAL AND ETHICAL ISSUES IN THE MANAGEMENT OF AGGRESSION AND VIOLENCE

Brodie Paterson and Cheryl Tringham

Introduction

There is at present very little educational guidance on the extent and limits of the authority afforded to health care professionals in the exercise of their duties towards clients. Professionals need to know the source of their authority, how far it extends and where to go for guidance if they are in doubt; otherwise, they may be forced to act on grounds of expediency or necessity without any clear principles to guide them. As a consequence, they may find themselves open to allegations of undue influence, professional misconduct, negligence or assault. In order to protect the public from the ill-informed professional, and the professional from litigation, a more comprehensive and realistic approach to the subject is, therefore, required.

The case for such knowledge is further strengthened by the changing context of care provision within which the nurse is expected to function, and the current trend and increasing public demand for professionals to be held accountable for their practice. If independent practitioners are to exercise mature judgement, formulating rational decisions for which they can be accountable, and at the same time function within a rapidly changing context of care, they must be aware of the professional, ethical and legal frameworks that shape nursing practice.

This chapter examines such frameworks and the ways in which they be should be utilised to formulate decisions about the application of force towards, and/or the restriction of liberty of, clients who present with aggressive and violent behaviour. Essentially the chapter is structured in two parts. The first part very briefly reconsiders the issue of epidemiology before going on to consider the legal position of employers and practitioners. The latter part of the chapter focuses on the ethical principle of autonomy, which currently has primacy in shaping the health care professional's practice. Autonomy will be examined specifically in relation to the delivery of care to those clients who present with aggressive and violent behaviour. The legal, ethical and professional sources of support for using this principle are identified, as are the consequences of failing to respect the client's autonomy.

Is exposure to violence a foreseeable event?

In considering aggression and violence from a legal perspective, involving a potential risk to staff health, it is necessary first to establish whether their occurrence in nursing is a 'foreseeable' event, that is, one that we can reasonably expect to happen (Dickson *et al.* 1993). Chapter 2 has established that research by the Health Services Advisory Committee (1987), Ryan and Postner (1993) and Stark *et al.* (1995) concurs in indicating that certain areas of nursing, namely services for people with a learning disability and challenging behaviour, accident and emergency units and acute mental health facilities, have a much higher frequency of serious incidents than other areas. It has also been established, however, that incidents can be expected to occur, albeit with a lower frequency, across nursing, midwifery and health visiting in a variety of settings from the medical, obstetric or care of elderly ward to the patient's or client's own home. It is thus undeniable that violence is a foreseeable event in many nursing work settings.

Is exposure liable to be harmful?

Second, it is necessary to establish the nature of the risk aggression and violence posed to nurses' welfare (MacKay 1994). Nurses are at risk both physically and psychologically as a consequence of exposure to aggression and violence (Engel and Marsh 1986). The threat to well-being arising from physical assault is generally recognised, and fatalities to nurses and other health care workers provide a salutary reminder of the potential seriousness of the issue, but as well as leading to the evident danger of physical harm, aggression and violence, can also produce psychological consequences. These can include increased stress levels (Whittington and Wykes 1992) and post-traumatic stress disorder (Mason 1991, Turnbull 1993). These can in turn have significant financial consequences for the organisation, which may arise through increased sickness and absence, decreased staff effectiveness or directly from legal action by the employee (Ishimoto 1984, Lanza and Milner 1989, Hunter and Carmel 1992). The nature of the relationship between staff sickness and absence and aggression and violence is, however, neither simple nor easy to determine (Rix 1987).

The issue of stress may not be a problem just in terms of nurses' health. There is an inverse relationship between excessive stress levels and the ability to perform effectively that can be demonstrated across a variety of situations. Excessive stress levels reduce cognitive efficiency and emotional control, and thus the ability to function effectively. Potentially violent situations are innately stressful, and increased stress levels relating to the repeated experience of what are often extremely difficult situations may inhibit the ability to practise effectively. They may even be a factor in increasing the risk of assault by nurses and care staff on clients (Breakwell 1989).

The law and employer liability

If violence is a foreseeable event in many areas of nursing (Stark *et al.* 1995), what are the legal implications of this? An employer who fails to comply with relevant health and safety provision may be guilty of a criminal offence, but civil actions for negligence cannot be brought on the basis of failure to observe health and safety legislation. The basis for the majority of civil actions is an alleged failure to observe a 'duty of care'. In civil cases, the plaintiff has to prove his case on 'balance of probabilities only', which contrasts with the standard of proof in criminal cases, which is 'beyond reasonable doubt'.

The tort of negligence (in failure to observe a duty of care) in civil law has been defined as:

a breach by the defendant of a legal duty to take reasonable care which results in damage being caused to the plaintiff. (Lyon 1994, p. 82)

The law of negligence requires that, in order for liability for injury to be established:

The defendant can be established to owe a legal duty of care to the plaintiff. (Miers and Shapland 1994)

The defendant has failed to observe this duty of care by falling below what could be reasonably expected of him. The concept is of a notional standard of care, and the test normally applied in medical negligence claims, for example, is what has become known as the Bolam test (Lyon 1994). It arises from the case of *Bolam* v. *Friern Hospital Management Committee* [1957] in which Bolam sued for damages for injuries sustained from the administration of electroconvulsive therapy (ECT) without the prior administration of a muscle relaxant. The view expressed by McNair was that that treatment should be considered lawful if it had been administered in accordance with the opinion of a responsible body of professional opinion. The existence of an opposing view is not adequate. In some circumstances, however, the court may decide to disregard this precedent if it believes that professional opinion and practice fall below the standard that may be reasonably expected in the circumstances (*Sidaway* v. *Board of Governors Bethlehem Royal Hospital* [1985]).

In Scotland, the test of negligence that would be applied is substantively different and involves consideration of whether a practitioner 'has been proved to be guilty of such failure as no practitioner of ordinary skill would be guilty of if acting with ordinary care' (*Hunter* v. *Hanley* [1955], s. 200):

The breach of the duty of care must have caused harm of the kinds that a court will compensate. (Carson 1996)

The injury was foreseeable and that the plaintiff was in a sufficiently proximate relationship with the negligent organisation or practitioner. (Carson 1996)

The issue of proximity relates to the degree to which the person causing the injury by his or her actions or failure to act was under the supervision of the defending organisation, or where the proximity or the identity of the claimant made potential injury to them highly likely (Miers and Shapland 1994).

Employers may thus be liable to prosecution and/or civil lawsuit if, by their actions or inactions and/or the actions or inactions of their employees, such actions breach statutory legislation or the common law standard of duty of care.

Example 4.1

A hospital Trust is being sued by a nurse, who had been working in its accident and emergency department, for compensation for physical injuries and associated psychological trauma that she alleges she sustained as a result of an assault by a patient. The nurse alleges that the Trust had failed to take reasonable steps to safeguard her welfare in providing her with a safe place of work. This had left her vulnerable to injury as a consequence of patient assault, and her employers had thus been negligent.

The defending Trust will be required to demonstrate:

that reasonable steps (likely to be interpreted as including policy development, risk assessment, training needs analysis, provision of training to identified competencies and necessary updating as well as the provision of alarms, security cameras and so on) had been taken to reduce the possibility of her experiencing injury.

or:

(a) that assault was not a foreseeable risk in the nurse's work environment
(b) that a reasonable body of professional opinion held that she did not require training in the management of violence
(c) that training would not have materially decreased the risk of her being assaulted and/or suffering injury in the course of an assault and, consequently thereof, that the failure to provide training did not materially contribute to her risk of experiencing injury.

Example 4.2

Client A, an in-patient in a mental health rehabilitation unit, assaults another client, B. Client B then attempts to sue the provider of his care for compensation for his injuries sustained as a consequence of that assault.

The defendant would have to demonstrate:

(a) that the assault was not foreseeable, for example that Client A the assailant had not previously committed acts of a similar nature

(b) or that the actions or inactions of members of staff providing care to both A and B in that environment did not fall below a reasonable standard
(c) or that, if they did, their actions did not materially contribute to the risk of the client being assaulted.

(There are of course a number of other defences in this instance, including potential provocation by B.)

Court discretion and the duty of care

The courts have the ultimate discretion to determine where a duty of care will be applied and may decide in some circumstances that imposing a duty of care is undesirable. In the case of *Hill* v. *Chief Constable of W. Yorkshire* [1988], the mother of one of the last victims of Peter Sutcliffe brought a case for negligence against the police. She alleged that they had conducted the investigation into the crimes committed by Peter Sutcliffe negligently and that her daughter had died because the failure by the police to act competently had materially contributed to the death of her daughter through their failure to arrest Peter Sutcliffe before he could commit further crimes. The House of Lords decided that to impose a duty of care in such circumstances was undesirable because it would have resulted in the police adopting 'unduly defensive practices' (Miers and Shapland 1994, p. 137), which would ultimately have affected their ability to fulfil their professional duties.

The law and the nurse

The way in which the law affects the actions of individual practitioners is in some respects similar to the way in which it affects their employers. They are affected by the statutory provisions of Health and Safety legislation and are required to exercise a duty of care in carrying out the duties and activities arising from their employment. They are, however, in a different position from their employers in that their direct interaction with the client requires them to have an awareness of other areas of statute and common law (particularly that relating to assault and unlawful detention). Professional nurses are also different in that they are required to adhere to the *Code of Professional Conduct* of their regulatory body, the United Kingdom Central Council for Nursing, Midwifery and Health Visiting (UKCC 1992), to work according to a set of ethical principles and to follow specific guidance and legislation with regard to their client group.

Practitioners must be aware that any restriction on the liberty or autonomy of an individual may, unless a lawful excuse for their use in a particular instance can be offered, become an offence. The potential criminal charges include *false imprisonment* and *assault and battery*.

False imprisonment

False imprisonment has been defined as 'an act of the defendant which directly and intentionally or negligently causes the confinement of the plaintiff within an area delimited by the defendant' (Brazier *Law of Torts*, p. 28, cited by Lyon 1994, p. 76).

Confinement includes any situation where an individual is prevented from leaving a building of any type, a hospital (including its grounds), a room, a vehicle, a specific area or even a chair. For confinement to be considered to have occurred, the restriction on liberty must be total, such that the client would risk injury if he or she tried to escape, or it would be unreasonable, because of the client's position, to expect him or her to try to escape. Using this definition, a variety of measures used that are the subject of professional controversy, such as 'Buxton' or tilt-back chairs (which restrict an individual's freedom of movement), cot sides, 'strong' clothing, arm splints, seclusion and some forms of medication can technically be considered to be 'false imprisonment'.

Example 4.3

Ryan, an adolescent with a severe learning disability and challenging behaviour who lives at home, has regular respite care every second weekend in a small, staffed group home. He is incontinent of faeces and can sometimes smear the faeces over himself and his surroundings. Without consultation with a clinical nurse specialist or clinical psychologist, the nurse in charge decides that Ryan's behaviour is 'attention seeking' and that it should be managed by 'time out'. Following any episode of smearing, Ryan should be placed in the bathroom on his own with the door held shut to prevent his escape.

In Example 4.3, as well as being unethical, it may well be that the nurse's behaviour has been unlawful, in that she could face a charge of false imprisonment for restricting Ryan's liberty by not allowing him to leave the bathroom.

Assault and battery

In English law, an assault is defined as 'any act of the defendant which directly and either intentionally or negligently causes the plaintiff immediately to apprehend a contact with his person' (Wilkinson et al. 1990). Battery is defined 'as any act of the defendant which directly and intentionally or negligently causes some physical contact with the plaintiff without the plaintiff's consent' (Brazier 1989, cited by Lyon 1994, p. 79). In both instances, the type of contact, whether actually experienced or feared, must clearly go beyond that liable to be experienced in everyday life.

In Scots law, assault is an attack on the person of another. It is a crime of intent. The slightest amount of force is enough, and there need be no actual injury; it cannot be committed recklessly or negligently. The unintentional infliction of personal injury is in certain circumstances criminal, but it is not an assault (Wilkinson et al. 1990)

Ethical principles and professional responsibilities

A knowledge of the law is important to any health care professional, but it is important that practitioners' decision-making processes are influenced by more than just a desire to avoid potential legal consequences: their decision-making and care should reflect an understanding of the principles of ethics.

The principle of autonomy

Many commentators (for example Downie and Calman 1987, Edwards 1996) emphasise the central importance of autonomy in health care ethics. Indeed, the value accorded the principle is reflected in contemporary health care practice, in which health care professionals are expected to acknowledge and respect client autonomy. Aitken and Tarbuck (1995) stress that nurses and other health care professionals must strive to promote rather than deny autonomy and that autonomy should be restricted only in certain circumstances. By autonomy is meant self-determination and self-rule, the capacity of an individual to act freely in accordance with a self-chosen plan. In other words, it is the ability of individuals to think and, on the basis of such thought, make decisions about their own welfare and future. Beauchamp and Childress (1994, p. 123) analyse autonomous action in terms of:

> normal choosers who act intentionally, with understanding, and without controlling influences that influence their action.

It is evident from this analysis that autonomous action is composed of a number of essential conditions; intention, understanding and independence from controlling influences. Furthermore, it should be noted that actions can be autonomous by degrees. To insist that all actions be fully autonomous, that is, be based on full understanding and be completely free from controlling influences, would be to set the standard for autonomous action so high that few, if any, individuals would ever achieve it. This is of importance as people's actions are rarely, if ever, fully autonomous. Furthermore, the presence of autonomy is for many the necessary and sufficient condition of 'personhood status', a status that confers upon its bearer access to human rights. Therefore, if the standard for autonomy were set at an ideal level, few if any would count as persons, and they would thus not have access to the corresponding rights that such status denotes.

It is widely recognised that possessing the capacity to demonstrate autonomous action is not the same as being respected as an autonomous agent. Being respected as an autonomous agent involves being treated in a manner that acknowledges one's right to make choices based on one's own personal values and beliefs, and also one's right to act on those choices.

Nurses and health care professionals have not only a moral duty to respect the autonomy of their clients, but also a professional and a legal duty to do so. This legal duty is evidenced in the requirement to obtain consent prior to the provision of treatment or care. The source of this legal duty is to be found in common law, which 'has long recognised the principle that every person has the right to have his bodily integrity protected against invasion by others' (Mason and McCall Smith 1991, p. 228), while the *Guidelines for Professional Practice* (UKCC 1996, p. 17) state that 'You must obtain consent before you can give treatment or care.'

Whereas most, if not all, of us would accept the idea that we should respect the autonomy of others, this acceptance is often not evidenced in the nurse practitioners' day-to-day practice.

Example 4.4

A client with a serious mental health problem is distressed and becoming increasingly agitated. De-escalation strategies have been attempted but have been unsuccessful. When the client is offered her prescribed as-required medication, she refuses. However, you, the senior registered nurse on duty, believe that it is in the client's best interests for her to take the medication in order to prevent a deterioration in her condition and to protect her and others from potential injury.

Example 4.4 outlines a situation in which the client makes a treatment choice that is at odds with that of the nurse, and which the latter considers not to be in the client's best interests. This can pose a very real dilemma for nurses. On the one hand, the nurse is charged with an obligation to act in the client's best interests, as evidenced in Clause 1 of the UKCC *Code of Professional Conduct* (1992), which asserts that the nurse must 'act always in a manner as to promote and safeguard the interests and well-being of patients and clients'. This duty to act in the client's best interests can, according to Edwards (1996, p. 69), be reasonably interpreted as a statement to the effect that the nurse is obliged to practise in accord with the obligations generated by the principle of beneficence. On the other hand, the nurse is charged with a duty to foster and develop client autonomy, as is evidenced in Clause 5 of the aforementioned code (UKCC 1992).

work in an open and co-operative manner with patients, clients... foster their independence and recognise and respect their involvement in the planning and delivery of care.

Thus, while Clause 1 promotes beneficence, Clause 5 strongly indicates that it is the duty of the nurse to 'foster' the autonomy of clients.

Here is a classic moral dilemma in nursing ethics, which is generated by a clash between obligations stemming from different moral principles, in this instance the principle of respect for autonomy and the principle of beneficence. Both of these principles, as noted previously, are cited in the UKCC *Code of Professional Conduct* (1992), which purports to be a framework for assisting nurses in the ethical aspects of their professional practice. However, as can be seen from this example, the Code assigns no relative weight to the demands of these principles when they conflict and consequently offers little help when a judgement has to be made. In this instance and indeed others, the Code, rather than providing guidance on which of these principles should take precedence in informing the nurse's judgement, results only in unhelpful pluralism, leading to intractable conflicts between principles and to conflicting moral injunctions.

If the principle of respect for autonomy is taken to be the first, highest-order principle, then in the situation described, the nurse's obligation is to respect the autonomous wishes of that client, regardless of her own personal opinion regarding the appropriateness of the client's decision. Example 4.4 illustrates that adherence to the principle of respect for persons may pose a number of difficulties to the nurse or other health care professional, as, while the principle asserts a broad, abstract obligation that is free from exceptive clauses, this respect is not absolute. In order to become a practical guide for action, the principle needs to specify the valid exceptions to the broad general rule. It is to these exceptions that we will now turn.

A conflict of interests

Respect for autonomy has only prima facie standing and can be overridden by competing moral considerations. The autonomy of an individual can be limited if the exercising of their autonomous action unnecessarily compromises the security needs of the individual in question or fails to take reasonable account of the autonomy of others. (At this juncture, only the latter will be explored; the former will be examined later in the text.) According to Beauchamp and Childress (1994), wide agreement exists that an individual's right of autonomy is often legitimately constrained by the rights of others. This may be evidenced by the fact that society currently legitimises certain forced medical interventions to serve what it considers to be important social goals, such as promoting public health, enforcing criminal law or otherwise promoting the safety and well-being of others (President's Committee 1983, cited in Kennedy and Grubb 1994, pp. 233–5). In illustrating this point, let us return to Example 4.4 above in which a distressed and increasingly agitated client refuses her prescribed as-required medication.

The previous experience of you, the nurse, with this particular client suggests that, if she does not take her medication at this point, her behaviour will escalate into violence towards other more vulnerable clients. Should the nurse still respect the client's wishes or disregard her expressed wishes and proceed to administer the medication in the absence of consent? While, as stated previously, society does legitimise certain forced medical interventions, the law may equally view any intervention forced on clients without their consent or against their expressed wishes as a crime or a civil wrong.

Ethically acceptable and legally defensible

Essentially, in order for the application of force and/or the restriction of liberty of adults to be considered legitimate, two principal criteria must be met (Gostin 1986), although it should also be noted that the overarching principle is always that no alternative to the use of force is available.

The two principal criteria identified by Gostin (1986) are as follows:

A legitimate reason to use force and/or restrict the liberty of an individual must exist.

The force and/or restriction utilised must be demonstrably reasonable.

Lawful excuse

According to Hoggett (1985, 1990), there exist five principal categories of legitimate reasons for the use of force and/or restriction of an individual's liberty:

■ *The prevention of a crime.* The English Criminal Law Act explicitly states that 'A person may use such force as is reasonable in the circumstances in the prevention of a crime' (reasonableness is examined below). This would potentially include any statutory offence, although for very minor offences, any use of force may be considered unreasonable.
■ *The prevention of a breach of the peace.* Lyon (1994, p. 89) defines a breach of the peace as a situation in which 'harm is done or likely

to be done to a person or in his presence, to his property: or harm is feared through an affray, riot, assault or other disturbance'.

■ *Self-defence*. While the law imposes a duty on any potential victim to retreat and escape, it also recognises that it may not always be possible to disengage. In the latter circumstances, the use of force and/or the restriction of liberty in self-defence is likely to be considered legitimate (Martin 1990).

■ *The restraint of a dangerous lunatic*. Under common law, there exists the power to detain the insane if their behaviour places their own or others' safety at risk. There is no suggestion that this is appropriate terminology – a modern interpretation of these concepts would generally include those individuals covered under the term 'mental disorder' used in both the Mental Health Act 1983 and the Mental Health (Scotland) Act 1984, which incorporates both those experiencing mental ill-health and those with learning disabilities (Hoggett 1990; Lyon 1994, p. 87).

■ *Exercise of statutory powers/duties*. In certain contexts, such as those mentioned above, the authority to use force may be derived from specific statute legislation.

With reference to Example 4.4 above, the nurse could administer the prescribed medication in the absence of the client's consent, and against her expressed wishes, if any of the aforementioned lawful excuses applied.

Nurses and other health care professionals must be aware that any application of force and/or restriction of the liberty or autonomy of an individual may, unless a lawful excuse for same can be forwarded, constitute a criminal or civil wrong (Miller 1991). The criminal charges that may result include those of false imprisonment, assault and, in English law, battery, all of which have previously been outlined in this chapter.

Reasonable force

Even where the law provides a potentially legitimate reason for the use of force, any force and/or restriction of an individual's liberty must be able to meet the criteria of 'reasonableness' (Gostin 1986). The notion of reasonableness is complex and can only, in any given instance, be absolutely determined by a court of law (Lyon 1994). Reasonableness in this context has, however, been defined as:

the force used should be no more than was necessary to accomplish the object for which it is allowed (so retaliation, revenge and punishment are not permitted) and second, the reaction must be in proportion to the harm which is threatened, in both degree and duration. (Dimond 1990)

A situation of imminent risk is one in which a nurse may be required to make split-second decisions concerning risks that have not been anticipated. It would seem likely that, if the degree of force used conforms to the principles previously set out, the courts would probably interpret it in such a way that there would be no criminal or civil liability.

Sometimes, however, situations may involve instances where the risk is either less immediate, for example an elderly person who wanders, or is occurring with such frequency that it can be anticipated. These kinds of situation need to be pre-planned and built into an individual care plan.

The questions the nurse or other health care professional must ask concerning Example 4.5 are:

Example 4.5

A frail elderly woman aged 83 who is experiencing dementia is being nursed in a general surgical ward following emergency surgery to pin a broken elbow after a fall at home. She is confused and disorientated, repeatedly trying to get out of bed despite an unstable gait. She vigorously strikes out at staff with her hands (including the limb that is in a cast) when they attempt to prevent her climbing out of bed or try to provide nursing care.

---

1. What are the risks to the client and others, including other clients and staff, from this lady's behaviour at this point, and should her behaviour continue? Can these risks be quantified?
2. What are the alternatives to the present management strategy, and what are the likely risks inherent in each alternative? Potential alternatives that could be explored are:

   ■ Could 'one-to-one' support be provided to allow the woman to wander safely under close supervision, negating the potential need for restraint?

■ Could her medication be reviewed with a view to short-term sedation?

If no other effective alternative to restraint appears to be available, the question of restraining the client either by manually holding her or by using some form of mechanical restraint to pin her might be considered. The risk of restraining, which has the potential to cause harm (Miles and Irvine 1992), should be considered against the risk of not restraining in deciding whether it is reasonable in this situation to physically restrain. The patient's relatives might be involved or consulted at this point.

It should be possible to demonstrate that all other alternatives have been considered and that restraint is the only method capable of minimising a significant risk to the client's and/or others' welfare. In addition, it should be possible to demonstrate that the risk associated with the use of the restraint employed, whether manual or mechanical, can be reasonably held to be less than that of not restraining.

Having considered the legally acceptable justifications for constraining an individual's right to autonomy, and the legal standard used to evaluate the appropriateness of the force utilised, we will now turn to another exception to the broad general rule of respecting the autonomy of others.

Autonomy status

As previously stated, despite the breadth of our obligations to respect autonomy, the principle has only prima facie standing and is not so broad that it covers non-autonomous persons. It is not possible to respect the autonomous nature of those who are not autonomous, that is, those who lack the necessary conditions of autonomous action: intent, understanding and freedom from controlling influences. The principle should not be used for those who cannot act in a sufficiently autonomous manner and cannot be rendered autonomous because they are immature or incompetent, or have been coerced or exploited. Thus, in respecting the autonomous wishes of our clients, the nurse must ascertain that their expressed wishes are truly autonomous, that is, that clients possess the necessary conditions of autonomy – intent, understanding and independence from controlling influences. When assessing the autonomy status of a given client, the nurse must pay cognisance to the following factors, any or all of which may interfere with the client's autonomy status.

Lack of understanding and involuntariness

Respecting autonomy requires more than an obligation of non-interference in the affairs of individuals. It also includes obligations to maintain an individual's capacity for autonomous choice and to allay fears and other conditions that may destroy or disrupt the individual's autonomous actions. In order to illustrate this point, let us return once again to Example 4.4. It may be that in the situation described here, the client in question is not in possession of the necessary knowledge upon which to form an autonomous choice regarding whether or not to accept the medication offered. Mill (1962) insisted that, when faced with the false or ill-considered views of others, we may sometimes be obligated to seek to persuade them of their misconceptions, and in this way actively strengthen their autonomous expression (Beauchamp and Childress 1994, p. 125). It is clear, therefore, that one demand created by the principle of respect for persons is that it denotes a corresponding duty on others to treat clients in a manner enabling them to act autonomously. Thus the nurse has a duty to provide clients with the knowledge necessary to enable them to make an informed and autonomous choice regarding their preferred course of action. Such knowledge can be gained both during and following information disclosure, the provision of which will facilitate understanding.

Support for this general demand of the principle of respect for persons is to be found in the following paragraphs from the *Guidelines for Professional Practice* (UKCC 1996):

> [Discuss] with them any proposed treatment or care so that they can decide whether to refuse or accept that treatment or care. This information should enable the patient or client to decide what is in their own best interests. (para. 20)

> You must make sure that all decisions are based on relevant knowledge. (para. 21)

> The patient or client can only make an informed choice if he or she is given clear information at every stage of care. (para. 22)

Indeed, the importance of the disclosure of information is evidenced throughout the guidance offered in the aforementioned document, as indeed are the legal repercussions of failing in one's duty to disclose the necessary information upon which clients can base their decisions with respect to treatment. These repercussions are allegations of negligence, or rarely, in exceptional cases, where the information disclosure was such that the client's consent could be said to have been obtained by deception, allegations of battery or civil assault in Scotland (UKCC 1996, para. 28). However, one issue not addressed in the UKCC guidance document (1996) is that of the quality, nature and extent of information disclosure that should be made to clients, although paragraph 23 does issue guidance in relation to the clarity of the language used (UKCC 1996).

This is a worrying oversight as a failure to look closely and analytically at the provision of advice and information to clients presents a considerable risk to client autonomy, and inadequate disclosure could negate the legal status of the client's consent. Failure to disclose adequate information upon which clients can base their treatment or care decisions may be interpreted as a manipulation of the clients' decision-making by the nurse or health care professional.

Manipulation

Of particular concern in the health care context is the withholding or distortion of information in order to affect the client's beliefs and decisions. Since it is the health care professional who has the information, he or she can determine the amount of information that the client will receive. According to Rumbold (1993), nurses or other health care professionals often claim to be allowing clients to make informed decisions about their treatment and care, while evidence suggests that they provide clients with only selected information. One possible example of such a practice is when the nurse or other health care professional outlines the various courses of treatment available to a particular client for a particular disorder but the information is presented in a manner in which there is a strong bias in favour of the nurse's or health care professional's preference. The outcome of such selective information disclosure means that the client will almost certainly elect for the course of action that the professional considers to be the best. Such behaviour may justly be criticised on two grounds: first, that it interferes with the client's voluntary choice, and second, that it interferes with the client's ability to make an informed decision, thus negating the client's consent.

According to the President's Committee on voluntariness in the decision-making process (1988, cited in Kennedy and Grubb 1994, p. 233), 'the client's participation in the decision-making process and ultimate decision regarding care must be voluntary'. A choice that has resulted from serious manipulation of an individual's ability to make an intelligent and informed decision is not the person's own free choice. This has long been recognised in law because, as stated above, a consent forced by threats or induced by fraud or misrepresentation is legally viewed as no consent at all, and the professional who obtains and acts on a consent obtained in this way may be subject to a charge of negligence, assault or battery. Furthermore, from the moral perspective, a consent obtained in such a manner is substantially involuntary and does not provide moral authorisation for treatment because it does not respect the client's dignity and may not reflect the aims of the client.

While it is acknowledged that it would be impossible to give a standard answer to the question of that which constitutes adequate information disclosure, given that such an answer would be dependent on individual clients and their circumstances, guidance on a legally acceptable test to measure the scope of necessary disclosure, and the situations in which it must, could or should be made, is available:

> the issue of whether non-disclosure in a particular case should be condemned as a breach of the [doctor's] duty of care is an issue to be decided primarily on the basis of expert [medical] evidence, applying the Bolam test. (Lord Bridge, cited in Kennedy and Grubb 1994, p. 185)

Thus, the test used to measure the adequacy of information disclosure is the same test that is used to measure the reasonableness of the actions of any professional person, namely the Bolam test:

> The test is the standard of the ordinary skilled man exercising and professing to have that special skill. A man need not possess the highest expert skill at the risk of being found negligent... it is sufficient if he exercises the skill of an ordinary competent man exercising that particular art. (*Bolam* v. *Friern Hospital Management Committee* [1957])

In Scotland, the test that may be applied is substantively different and involves consideration of whether a practitioner 'has been proved to be guilty of such failure as no practitioner of ordinary skill would be guilty of acting with ordinary care' (*Hunter* v. *Hanley* [1995]).

Thus, according to the Bolam principle, the central element in assessing the quality of your own information disclosure, as a nurse, is whether or not other nurses, as representatives of a responsible body of professional opinion, would or would not have done as you did. The legal position in Scotland may differ, in that the criteria are that no other practitioner would have done what you did, that is, manipulate and/or withhold certain information from a client.

Whereas, as previously stated, understanding will be facilitated by the provision of information and knowledge, another necessary component of understanding is competence – the ability to undertake a cost/benefit analysis and, on the basis of the same, to arrive at a decision.

Competence

Another factor to be considered in the nurse's assessment of the client's autonomy status is the client's competence to make a decision. In practice, questions regarding a client's competence rarely emerge unless there is disagreement between the parties. So long as the client concurs with the nurse's or other health care professional's recommendations, the client's competence to understand, to decide and to consent to treatment is rarely examined. It is when there is conflict between what the client's wishes and the doctor's judgement about what serves that client's best interests that an inquiry into the client's competence is provoked.

Attempts to elucidate the notion of competence are fraught with difficulties, but there is, according to Beauchamp and Childress (1994, p. 134), a single core meaning, that is, 'the ability to perform a task'. However, the criteria of particular competencies are relative to the specific task or decision to be undertaken; for example, the criteria for someone's competence to stand trial, to manage their finances, to drive a car or to manage their personal welfare are radically different. Possessing the competence to decide is, therefore, relative to the particular decision to be made, and incompetence with regard to one decision-making area of life does not imply incompetence in all areas. Thus an individual may at the same time be considered competent for some legal purposes and incompetent for others. Furthermore, while an individual's competence in a given task can range from full mastery through various levels of proficiency to complete inability, for practical and policy reasons, a threshold level of competence is required. Below this threshold, a person with a certain level of ability is deemed to be incompetent. In this way, two basic classes, competent and incompetent, are created, into which individuals can be sorted, thus distinguishing those individuals whose decisions should be respected from individuals whose decisions need not or should not be respected.

While a general presumption exists that adults are competent to make their decisions, this is a presumption that can be rebutted. To be considered competent to make a decision, the individual must be able to comprehend 'the material information, to make a judgement about the information in light of his or her values, to intend a certain outcome, and to freely communicate his or her wishes to caregivers' (Beauchamp and Childress 1994, p. 135). Unfortunately, the assessment of competence raises many troublesome questions concerning the validity and reliability of the assessment process (see, for example, Buchanan and Brock 1989, Kennedy and Grubb 1994, and Beauchamp and Childress 1994, for an analysis of the rival standards and tests). What is clear from the legal evidence to date is that the status approach to the determination of competency has been rejected. This is a manifestly subjective and unjust approach that utilises the client's status, for example 'learning disabled' or 'mentally ill', as the sole criterion for determining the client's decision-making capacity. Instead, the law favours a notion of competence centred on understanding, as is evidenced in case law (Gillick cited in Kennedy and Grubb 1994, p. 118), and the Age of Legal Capacity Act (Scotland) 1991, which gives statutory expression to the decision in Gillick. According to Kennedy and Grubb (1994, p. 123), the most important factor in determining competence is that 'the health care professional, both as a matter of ethics and law, has a duty to behave with integrity and be satisfied that the criteria deemed relevant to determine capacity are present in the particular case'.

Consider again Example 4.4, in which the client is distressed and becoming increasingly agitated. Would it make any difference in terms of what the nurse legally could or could not do if the client were competent or incompetent? If the client were deemed to be competent to make her own treatment choices, the justification for overriding her expressed wishes could only be made by reference to the lawful excuses outlined previously, and the force utilised in the administration of the treatment must meet the standard of reasonableness. If, however, the client were deemed to be incompetent to make her own treatment decisions, the nurse could appeal to additional legal principles (additional to the lawful excuses already cited) to justify the use of force and/or restriction of liberty.

The law has long recognised that there are those who, through mental incapacity, are incapable of making their own treatment choices but pose no threat to others and are, as such, not subject to the legal provisions that justify the use of forced treatment. Essentially, the law adopts two approaches to such individuals, the approach selected depending on the nature of the individual's mental incapacity.

Substituted judgement approach

An autonomy-based approach, in terms of any treatment or care provided, is effectively directed toward the higher goal of restoring the client's already compromised autonomy. The use of this approach is restricted to those clients who have had and/or are expected to have once again a meaningful degree of autonomy through which to exercise decision-making (Mason and McCall Smith 1991, p. 393). When this approach is utilised, the question being asked regarding the propriety of the planned treatment is: Would the client, were he in possession of his rationality, consent to the treatment proposed? If the answer to this question is yes, the planned treatment can proceed in the absence of consent. If, however, the answer is no, an alternative course of action should be sought.

According to Mason and McCall Smith (1991, pp. 393–4), it is 'philosophically impossible' to utilise the substituted judgement for those clients who have never possessed and/or never will possess the necessary degree of autonomy through which to exercise decision-making, for example those whose mental incapacity is the product of a permanent condition such as learning disability. In such cases, it is thought to be more appropriate to adopt an approach based on 'best interests'.

Best interests approach

When considering any treatment or care provided, a beneficence-based approach is effectively directed toward a goal, which is not necessarily sought by the client but which is intended to promote that which is best for that particular client and which protects him or her from harm. When this approach is utilised, the question being asked regarding the propriety of the planned treatment is:

Will the proposed treatment serve the client's best interests and protect him or her from potential harm?

The best interests approach has been criticised on various grounds, one of which relates to the difficulties encountered in the determination of that which constitutes the best interests of another person. In addition, the Scottish Law Commission (1991, p. 110) criticised the best interests approach on the grounds that it was too vague and, as a consequence, allowed 'too much discretion and [gave] insufficient guidance'.

Despite these acknowledged difficulties, the courts have increasingly relied on this approach to justify the non-consensual treatment of those who are deemed incompetent. The courts themselves acknowledge the difficulties inherent in the application of this approach and, in determining the best interests of others, appeal to considerations of what most people in society consider to be the right or reasonable thing to do in the circumstances; this is what is known as the reasonable person standard.

One case illustrating the application of the best interests approach in treatment decisions for the mentally incapacitated is the case of In Re F (Mental Patient: Sterilisation) [1989]. The case concerned a 36-year-old woman with a learning disability who was described as being unable to express herself in words but capable of indicating her likes and dislikes. Concern for F's well-being arose as a consequence of a relationship that she had formed with a male resident. The exact nature of the relationship was never established, although it was felt that it probably involved sexual intercourse or something close to it. The staff of the hospital in which F resided, and her mother, were concerned at the possibility of pregnancy, and as a consequence they decided that F should be sterilised; this was felt to be the only method of contraception that would be both effective and feasible in F's case. As F could not provide a valid consent to the operation because of her mental disability, and because in English law no-one could consent on her behalf, F's mother sought a declaration from the court, to the effect that such an operation would not amount to an unlawful act by reason only of the absence of F's consent.

This case established two points relevant to the issue of the non-consensual treatment of those who are mentally incapacitated. First, treatment that was considered to be in an incompetent client's best interests could be given without his or her consent. Second, the case established that the test of whether the proposed treatment was in the client's best interests was to be determined by reference to the

Bolam principle. Thus, if the proposed treatment is in accordance with a practice accepted as proper by a responsible body of professional opinion, skilled in the particular form of treatment in question, the treatment will be considered to be in the client's best interests (*Bolam* v. *Friern Hospital Management Committee* [1957]). To put this another way, 'If a doctor (professional) can show that a number of his peers would reach a similar view to his, this would be enough to make his assessment of what was in a patient's best interests valid and lawful' (Kennedy 1992, p. 398).

The Bolam test 'was originally formulated in the context of whether doctors had been negligent in carrying out treatment. Arguably, it is not appropriate for deciding whether or not treatment should be given' (Scottish Law Commission 1991, p. 106). Indeed, questions have subsequently arisen about whether the Bolam test was sufficient to perform the task to which it was set in this context, because to say that it is not negligent to carry out a particular form of treatment does not mean that the treatment is in the individual's best interests. If one were to extrapolate this test to the cases under review here, the non-consensual treatment of clients who are mentally incapacitated, the result would be as follows: To determine whether treatment was really in the client's best interests, best interests would be measured by reference to the Bolam principle, that is, against whether the proposed treatment was in accordance with a practice accepted as proper by a responsible body of professional opinion skilled in the particular form of treatment in question. If the answer was yes, treatment would be considered to be in the client's best interests. In other words, the client's best interests would be answered and analysed by reference to Bolam.

As Brazier (1990, p. 25) points out, 'Judicial intervention on this basis does little more than protect [the mentally incapacitated] from the complete maverick whom none of his colleagues would back in his decision'. Furthermore, the Bolam test has been criticised on the basis that it gives undue weight to professional opinions and accepted practice (Shaw 1990). This is probably the most serious consequence of utilising the Bolam principle to evaluate the propriety of treatment decisions for clients who are mentally incapacitated, primarily because non-consensual treatment may be considered to be acceptable professional practice, and could as such be considered to be in the client's best interests on the basis of Bolam. If the Bolam test were to be extrapolated from the specific issue of sterilisation to the issue of the non-consensual treatment of clients who are mentally incapacitated, the profound question of the permissibility of enforcing treatment on such clients would be reduced to a question of professional opinion. If this were to be the case, the preservation and protection of the rights of those who are mentally incapacitated, the most vulnerable members of society, would be handed over to health/social care professionals.

Perhaps the use of the Bolam principle in assessing the best interests of those who are mentally incapacitated is simply a reflection of the attitudes of others to such devalued groups, 'For is it imaginable that any other group of people could have their best interests re-stated as merely the right not to have others make negligent decisions in relation to them' (Carson 1989, p. 372). The nub of concern here is that the best interests test should be used to facilitate a more objective enquiry into wider considerations rather than a simple, rudimentary enquiry of fact into whether a body of professionals, not necessarily a majority, would consider non-treatment to be appropriate.

Conclusion

While the principle of respect for persons is generally accepted as having primacy in contemporary health care practice, this chapter has highlighted some of the difficulties that strict adherence to this principle may present for health care professionals in their day-to-day practice with clients. However, given the philosophical, legal and professional value accorded to the principle, professionals should not be forced into submission by such difficulties.

Since nurses and health care professionals are required to practise in a society that appears increasingly orientated towards litigation, both they and their employers should be concerned to ensure that they are fully aware of what the law requires and allows them to do when faced with an aggressive or violent client. Ensuring good practice in this difficult and demanding area requires a knowledge of the professional, ethical and legal principles that underpin professional practice. Utilising these principles, a framework can be devised that practitioners can use to assess the propriety of the potential use of any force. While it is not necessary for every practitioner to be expected to acquire and maintain an in-depth understanding of this specialist area of knowledge, for those involved in those areas of practice where restraint and/or the restriction of liberty occur with regularity, such knowledge should be regarded as essential.

List of cases

Bolam *v.* Friern Hospital Management Committee [1957] 2 ALL ER.
Gillick *v.* West Norfolk and Wisbech Area Health Authority [1986] AC 112, [1985] 3 ALL ER 402.
Hill *v.* Chief Constable of W. Yorkshire [1988] 2 WLR 1049.
Hunter *v.* Hanley [1955] SLT 213 @217 in Re F (Mental Patient: Sterilisation) [1989] 2 WLR 1025.
Sidaway *v.* Board of Governors Bethlehem Royal Hospital [1985] AC 871, per Lord Bridge.

References

Aitken F. and Tarbuck P. (1995) Practical ethical and legal aspects of caring for the assaultive client. In Stark C. and Kidd B. (eds) *Management of Violence and Aggression In Health Care,* Gaskell/Royal College of Psychiatrists, London.
Age of Legal Capacity Act (Scotland) (1991) London, HMSO.
Beauchamp T.L. and Childress J.F. (1994) *Principles of Biomedical Ethics,* 4th edn, London, Oxford University Press.
Brazier M. (1989) *Clerk and Linsell on Torts,* 16th edn, London, Sweet & Maxwell.
Brazier M. (1990) Sterilisation: down the slippery slope? *Professional Negligence,* **6**: 25.
Breakwell G. (1989) *Facing Physical Violence,* London, British Psychological Society.
Buchanan A.E. and Brock D.W. (1989) *Deciding for Others: The Ethics of Surrogate Decision Making,* Cambridge, Cambridge University Press.
Carson D. (1989) The sexuality of people with learning difficulties, *Journal of Social Welfare Law,* (6): 355–72.
Carson D. (1996) Risking legal repercussions. In Kemshall H. and Pritichard J. (eds) *Good Practice In Risk Assessment,* London, Jessica Kingsley.
Dickson R., Cox T., Leather P., Beale D. and Farnsworth B. (1993) Violence at work, *Occupational Health Review,* **46**: 22–4.
Dimond B. (1990) *Legal Aspects of Nursing,* London, Prentice-Hall.
Downie, R.S. and Calman K.C. (1987) *Healthy Respect,* London, Faber & Faber.
Edwards S.D. (1996) *Nursing Ethics: A Principle-based Approach.* London, Macmillan.
Engel F. and Marsh S. (1986) Helping the employee victim of violence in hospitals, *Hospital and Community Psychiatry,* **37**: 159–62.
Gostin L. (1986) *Institutions Observed: Towards a New Concept of Secure Provision in Mental Health,* London, King Edward's Hospital Fund for London.
Health Services Advisory Committee (1987) *Violence to Staff in the Health Service,* London, HMSO.

Hoggett B. (1985) Legal aspects of secure provision. In Gostin L. (ed.) *Secure Provision*, London, Tavistock.

Hoggett B. (1990) *Mental Health Law*, 3rd edn, London, Sweet & Maxwell.

Hunter J. and Carmel H. (1992) The cost of staff injuries from inpatient violence, *Hospital and Community Psychiatry*, **43**(6): 586–8.

Ishimoto W. (1984) Security management for health care administrators. In Turner J.T. (ed.) *Violence in the Medical Care Setting: A Survival Guide*, Aspen, CO, Aspen Publications.

Kennedy I. (1992) *Treat Me Right*, Oxford, Clarendon.

Kennedy I. and Grubb A. (1994) *Medical Law: Text with Materials*, 2nd edn, London, Butterworths.

Lanza M.L and Milner J. (1989) The dollar cost of patient assault, *Hospital and Community Psychiatry*, **34**: 44–7.

Lyon C. (1994) *Legal Issues Arising from the Care, Control and Safety of Children with Learning Disabilities who also Present Severe Challenging Behaviour*, Mental Health Foundation, London.

MacKay C. (1994) Violence to health care professionals : a health and safety perspective. In Whykes T. (ed.) *Violence and Health Care Professionals*, London, Chapman & Hall.

Martin A. (1990) The case for self defence, *Health and Social Service Journal*, **88**: 697.

Mason J. and McCall Smith A. (1991) *Law and Medical Ethics*, 3rd edn, Edinburgh, Butterworths.

Mason P. (1991) Violent Trends, *Nursing Times*, **87**(21): 57–8.

Mental Health Act (England and Wales) (1983) London, HMSO.

Mental Health Act (Scotland) (1984) London, HMSO.

Miers D. and Shapland J. (1994) Compensation and the criminal justice system. In Whykes T. (ed.) *Violence and Health Care Professionals*, London, Chapman & Hall.

Miles S.H. and Irvine P. (1992) Deaths caused by physical restraints, *Gerontologist*, **32**(6): 762–6.

Mill J.S. ([1863] 1962) Utilitarianism. In Wainock M. (ed.) *Utilitarianism*, London, Fontana.

Miller R. (1991) Hitting back, *Nursing Times*, **87**(5): 57–8.

President's Committee (1983) *Making Health Care Decisions*: Report.

Rix G. (1987) Staff sickness and its relationship to violent incidents on a regional secure psychiatric ward, *Journal of Advanced Nursing*, **12**: 223–8.

Rumbold G. (1993) *Ethics in Nursing Practice*, London, Baillière Tindall.

Ryan J. and Postner E.C. (1993) Results of a survey into violence in nursing, *Nursing Times*, **91**(50): 57–61.

Scottish Law Commission (1991) *Mentally Disabled Adults: Legal Arrangements for Managing their Welfare and Finances*. Discussion Paper No. 94, Edinburgh, Scottish Law Commission.

Shaw J.S. (1990) Sterilisation of mentally handicapped patients: judges rule OK? *Medical Law Review*, **53**: 91.

Smith J.C. and Hogan B. (1988) *Criminal Law*, 6th edn, London: Butterworths.

Stark C., Paterson B. and Kidd B. (1995) Incidence of assaults on staff in the NHS, *Nursing Times*, **3**: 20.

Turnbull J. (1993) Victim support, *Nursing Times*, **89**(23): 33–4.

UKCC (1992) *Code of Professional Conduct*, London, UKCC.

UKCC (1996) *Guidelines for Professional Practice*, London, UKCC.

Whittington R. and Wykes T. (1992) Staff strain and social support in a psychiatric hospital following assault by a patient, *Journal of Advanced Nursing*, **17**(4): 480–5.

Wilkinson A.B., Wilson W.A., Hope J.A.D., MacLean R.N.M and Paton A. (1990) *Gloag and Hendersons Introduction to the Law of Scotland*, 8th edn, p. 823, Edinburgh, Green & Son.

5

VERBAL ABUSE

Rob Wondrak

Introduction

Verbal abuse is a problem that can confront all health care professionals in day-to-day practice. Studies into the abuse of professionals have emphasised the stressful effects of non-physical violence and have shown that it is often the most inexperienced members of various professions who are in the front line (Cox 1987, Health and Safety Commission 1987). The group of staff who are particularly at risk has been found to be student nurses. In the study conducted by the Health and Safety Commission (1987), the highest incidence of aggression was of verbal abuse, and, in a 12-month period, 4 out of 10 students who responded in the study had been the victims of verbally abusive behaviour. The incidence of aggression directed against staff has been increasing within the health care system (Whitman *et al.* 1976, Lion and Reid 1983, Fisher 1985).

This chapter will begin by briefly examining the psychology of verbal aggressiveness and review some of the main literature in this area. The second part will then examine some methods and techniques for dealing with verbal abuse.

During the past few years, there has been considerable discussion about the level of aggressiveness in therapeutic practice. Numerous articles have explored the issues of physical aggression and abuse, but little information is available about verbal abuse itself (Cox 1987).

Buss (1961) defined aggression as a response that delivers pain to others. This usually refers to physical abuse but can clearly also mean verbal abuse. The term 'aggression' is a word from the vernacular language that researchers have attempted to use scientifically, and, the term could, therefore, do with some clarification (Tedeschi 1983). The word 'aggression' applies to a wide variety of behaviours varying between numerous dimensions. For example, Buss (1961) has proposed three dimensions of aggressiveness: physical–verbal, active–passive and direct–indirect. Other writers have explored the issue of aggression as being a dynamic rather than a fixed entity. They argue that whether a given act is aggressive or not depends upon the behavioural norms for the situation and whether or not the act is justified (Caminski et al. 1984).

Aggression is a universal phenomenon, and the term is used in common, everyday parlance. Writers have, therefore, criticised attempts to use the term in a scientific sense in the studies. Tedeschi (1983) has proposed that the term be redefined as 'coercive power', whereby the main measure of the aggressive act is as a form of influence that uses force.

It is only during the past 10 years that the literature has differentiated between physical and verbal aggression (Cox 1987, Wondrak 1989). The topic has usually been treated in a generic way by writers. It is clearly important to differentiate between the two as there is evidence that impulsive physical aggression begins with verbal threats or abuse. This can then escalate into physical attack, such as 'shaking or pushing' (Berkowitz 1962), as a coercive form of interpersonal communication. For the purposes of clarity, verbal abuse is defined here as any expressed aggression or hostile verbal attack directed against any other individual. Verbal aggression consists of attacking a person's self-concept and/or their position on a topic and as such is obviously a barrier to any rational intervention (Remland 1982). It is, therefore, very important for practitioners to learn how to deal with protagonists without escalating their hostility.

There currently seems to be little information available to assist practitioners in dealing effectively with verbal abuse or hostility from clients. Most of the attempts to collect statistics and information on violent behaviour by hospitalised patients, particularly in psychiatry, have only occurred during the past two decades. Kalogerakis (1971) was one of the first authors to start collecting statistics on violent patients and discovered that most of the literature dealt mainly with physical aggression. In 1981, Bernstein surveyed over 450 practitioners in psychology, psychiatry, social work, marriage and family counselling (Bernstein 1981). Of all of these, 14 per cent indicated that they had been assaulted, 36 per cent had been threatened by patients, and psychiatrists were both more fearful of assault and more frequently assaulted than any other group. A survey of 300 independent practitioners revealed that 81 per cent had experienced at least one incident of a patient's physical attack, verbal abuse or other harassment in their practice, verbal abuse being the most frequently reported event. The author of this report drew attention to the issue of verbal abuse and argued that, although episodes did not seem as frightening as physical assault, it was clearly stressful, and she thus included specific questions about verbal abuse in her survey (Tyron 1986). This particular study also found that women were less likely than men to experience verbal abuse from their patients; however, most incidents occurred in work with adult male patients. Most practitioners also reported a moderate amount of fear associated with such incidents, female therapists feeling particularly more at risk. The more frightened the therapist seemed to be by the incident, the more likely he or she was to alter future patient selection or therapeutic approach (Tyron 1986).

Verbal abuse in nursing

During the past few years, researchers have focused on the problem of verbal abuse in nursing practice. The old adage 'Sticks and stones may break my bones, but names will never hurt me' is quoted by Curtin (1980) in the beginning of an editorial regarding verbal violence. Curtin maintains that this adage is clearly untrue, the recipients often remaining very upset.

Several studies have attempted to explore the link between gender and power existing within relationships. Reakes (1981) explores the relationship between abuse and sexism, describing the lack of concern about verbal abuse in nursing because, she argues, there is an implicit support for the patriarchal system, which emphasises nursing in a sexist way. Reakes compares the issues of the abused child, an image of the innocent vulnerability that the child creates, which can then have the effect of increasing feelings of anger in the abuser. This is linked with the image of the abused nurse and the nurse's inability to control and direct the profession that primarily arises from female sex role issues.

Reakes suggests that some nurse abuse may arise because the 'nurse victim' may not fit the stereotype that patients (and male colleagues) often have of the female nurse:

Female occupations are considered inferior to males and women are not expected to be successful. Women who work primarily with male workers and try to influence the male work group are considered different and are usually ignored. (Reakes 1981, p. 9)

She proposes the exploration of female sex issues in a formal and organised way in nursing in order to facilitate a better understanding of control and autonomy of issues, which will equip the nurse with a better ability to deal with these situations.

Continuing on this theme, other writers have agreed that the expectations of women in patriarchal systems can lead to difficulties when a woman does not conform to the role assigned. For example, Torres (1981) found that, in the university setting, a woman was often considered to be an outlaw if she did not conform to the role assigned to her by a largely patriarchal system.

Gordon and Green (1981) have discussed a successful workshop for registered nurses on understanding the impact of female sexual stereotyping in health care practice. They urge educators of nursing to break down sexual barriers by reinforcing new models of behaviour that are not traditional female-conforming behaviours.

More recently, interest in this area has attempted to explore links with 'oppressed group' behaviour. Cox (1991) argues that this concept could well apply to nurses, for whom the result of oppression is a form of institutionalised helplessness leading to poor self-regard.

Chitty and Maynard (1986) have described how patients often avoid closeness by behaving antagonistically in such encounters, including using sarcasm, making sexual comments, touching, aggressive questioning about personal matters and forgetting 'important aspects of self care'. Patients may also point out nurses' errors or comment on the nurses' problems. Chitty and Maynard have suggested that interventions in such situations should centre around the three basic issues of:

1. Trust
2. Security
3. Control.

There tends to be a general view in health care practice, particularly in nursing, that is linked to the adage 'Everyone must go through it; it is something that I have to cope with.' According to Kohnke (1981), this may be a key ethic in nursing. Developing this theme, Kohnke also draws parallels with the abuse cycle and compares the dynamics involved in child abuse with those occurring in nurse abuse. Parents who set unrealistic demands and expectations for themselves and their children experience poor self-images and low self-esteem, frustration and tensions that can culminate in child abuse. The cycle of abuse is perpetuated from generation to generation. Kohnke examines similarities between the parent abuse role and those which continue in nursing practice and seem to be perpetuated from 'generation to generation' of nurse graduates.

The report referred to above by the Health and Safety Commission (1987), which studied violence in the health service, found that the highest incidence of aggression reported was that of verbal abuse. In a 12-month period, 4 out of 10 students who responded to this study had been on the receiving end of some verbal attack. Student nurses were found to be in a particularly vulnerable position and were likely to be the recipients of anger or hostility. This vulnerability may be a result of their front-line position or of their lack of skill and experience in dealing with such patients. Another important factor may be the lack of any instruction in the handling of such situations in their educational programmes. Duldt (1981) has argued that health care professions frequently encounter anger in their day-to-day work and that the effects of anger have not been studied because anger is so common. Duldt suggests that nurses feel guilt associated with anger and, therefore, cannot deal effectively with anger when it is expressed towards them. She suggests that a general 'anger-dismay syndrome' develops (Duldt 1982). As a solution to this, she argues for the effective use of confrontation and the assertiveness techniques to be taught to nurses, as a method of coping with angry confrontations.

A fairly detailed analysis of verbal abuse took place in West Texas, carried out by Cox (1987). Cox looked at four main areas:

1. The incidence of verbal abuse
2. The incidence of verbal abuse on nursing turnover rates
3. The identification of the main source of verbal abuse in nursing practice
4. The methods used by nurses to respond to verbal abuse.

Cox concluded that verbal abuse is so prevalent that 'it is surprising that any of us stay in nursing!'

Of the staff nurses in Cox's study, 82 per cent reported the experience of verbal abuse in their practice. The survey revealed that nurses initially start to use assertiveness techniques but very frequently and quickly resort to avoidance techniques. Cox also found that at least 16–18 per cent of registered nurse turnover was due to verbal abuse. Importantly, medical staff were found to be the most common sources of abuse for 78 per cent of the staff nurses in her study.

The next most frequent source of verbal abuse for both staff nurses and other senior staff was patients' relatives. This study clearly highlights not only the intense problems in the welfare of the people concerned, but also the significant management and manpower implications of the findings. It seems vital that more research is conducted to refine the variables influencing the incidence of and success in dealing with verbal abuse.

The psychology of verbal aggressiveness

It is important to make a distinction between aggressiveness that is damaging and negative, and aggression that can be constructive and positive. Not all expressed anger is unhelpful. Expletives and verbally aggressive utterances can be very cathartic and can lead to an improved state of mind once the abusive term has been stated to those we feel may have done us harm. The verbal expletive is commonly an expression of verbal aggressiveness directed towards totally inanimate objects and does little harm. Consider our comments to the hammer when we hit our own thumb, or to the piece of furniture that we inadvertently kick with our toes. All this can be very helpful, and the expression of anger can often facilitate and improve communication and satisfaction. Verbal abuse, although it may seem very unlikely, can in some instances be a measure of intimacy or of an increased understanding and empathy between people. It can become destructive and negative if it produces the dissatisfaction occurring when at least one person in a dyad feels less favourable as a result of the intervention and the quality of the relationship is seriously affected (Infante 1987). Thus it may at times be sensible to encourage the expression of anger rather than to allow strong feelings to be bottled up and eventually erupt in a more violent and less containable way. Unfortunately, most nurse education programmes have not really addressed this area very effectively. The result is that patients are often left to cope alone with their strong or passionate feelings, the staff unwittingly colluding in the development of potentially violent outbursts. Verbal abuse and the expression of anger are related to an inability to use language adequately to express need.

Infante (1987) makes an interesting distinction between physical and verbal, or 'symbolic', aggression that occurs within the context of interpersonal relations. Physical aggression, he argues, involves using one's body, or an extension of the body, to apply force to dominate, defeat or control. Symbolic aggression, however, is used principally as a channel to dominate or destroy the person's self-concept. Assertiveness, as opposed to aggressiveness, may be viewed as a constructive form of symbolic aggressiveness in the context of interpersonal relations. A distinction can also be made between argumentativeness and aggressiveness. Argumentativeness may be the ability to present or defend positions relevant to a particular issue and to attack the positions that other people take (Infante and Rancer 1982). Argumentativeness may be considered to be a subset of assertiveness. The literature on the topic of assertiveness is fairly substantial and is beyond the scope of this particular chapter. Any reader wishing to follow this up further is referred to Infante's chapter 'Aggressiveness' in McCroskey and Daly (1987).

Psychology of the 'victim'

It was suggested above that the expression of verbal directness is also a feature of the level of intimacy that exists between people. We tend to shout and express our real feelings to individuals around us whom we trust. In other words, we save our angry exclamations for partners or friends, people for whom we have some awareness of the response we are likely to get back. While many instances of verbal abuse may be purely spontaneous and nothing to do with the possible relationship between the parties involved, it is worth considering this possibility further.

Wondrak (1989) cites a study that was carried out in Oxford on 115 respondents who were staff in the local Mental Health Unit, where 20 per cent of the respondents indicated that impulsive or spontaneous acts of verbal abuse had emerged with 'key' individuals being the victims, and these individuals often reported dealing with verbal abuse fairly often in their working lives. Thus in situations other than the impulsive outpourings of someone disinhibited through drugs or alcohol, we unconsciously choose people who we think will be able to 'contain' and manage our anger. Emphasis must, of course, be made to the reality that many of the abusive situations that confront all health care staff are related to drugs or alcohol intoxication. It is very difficult to be able to manage such situations, and caution is required. However, there is the possibility that, in many situations involving verbal hostility or abuse, the patients may in some instances be choosing individual practitioners with whom they feel *safe* to express their frustrations and feelings.

Another consideration highlighted by this study was that the staff who seemed to be able to define or use a clear theoretical model were able to tolerate the effects of the verbal abuse much better. For example, some of the staff cited the use of psychological theories underlying their practice. One particular respondent stated that having a 'psychodynamic' understanding helped her to view the behaviour less as a personal attack and enabled a more effective exploration of the underlying issues. Perhaps having some tools to work with provides the practitioner with some defence. It, therefore, becomes necessary for the practitioner to develop skills in discriminating those times to engage a protagonist and those times to leave well alone. Both are an indication of skill!

Methods of dealing with verbal abuse

Few articles have attempted to identify specific techniques of dealing with verbal abuse. Sandford (1985) believes that the strain placed upon nurses by verbal abuse is greater than that placed on any other occupational group because nurses spend at least 8 hours a day with patients and others who verbally attack them. She suggests some approaches, such as acknowledging the attacker's right to his or her viewpoint, questioning in an attempt to understand the person's anger, setting limits and keeping cool under pressure as methods of helping nurses to deal with episodes of verbal abuse.

Self and Viau (1980) have suggested four steps for helping the patient to alleviate anger:

1. The identification of signs of anger
2. The acceptance and acknowledgement of the patient's anger
3. The exploration of the patient's anger
4. Channelling the anger.

There are a number of basic prerequisites that are important to understand before considering the effectiveness of any technique of dealing with hostility or anger. First, it is important that the practitioner starts with *him* or *herself*. This means examining carefully and critically his or her own ways of dealing with anger and embarrassment.

Personal defensiveness

If we know the ways in which we are likely to react when provoked, it can help considerably in anticipation of the event. There is often a great deal of indignity and embarrassment caused by some verbal assault, and the otherwise competent practitioner is rendered speechless and then very defensive. This is the critical time, and it often leads to needless retaliation and escalation. An example of this from the author's own experience was of a very competent nurse who could deal effectively with many situations in a calm, assured and confident way until one day an angry patient criticised the nurse's big nose. The result was a complete deflation and collapse of individual self-esteem and, in a very embarrassed way, the nurse withdrew, totally upset for the rest of the day.

It thus becomes important to examine critically our own 'Achilles heel', the vulnerable parts of our own psychological make-up, perhaps talking through such fears and anxieties with a trusted colleague. It is sometimes surprising how individuals can 'home in' on what may be a particular area of discomfort.

Brammer (1979) suggests that the presence of the following six characteristics are important in the ability to cope with assaults:

1. *An awareness of self-values* (it is important to be personally reflective, examine and develop a keener sense of self-awareness)
2. *The ability to analyse one's own feelings*
3. *The ability to influence and act as a model to others*
4. *Altruism* (the ability to work for others irrespective of the rewards)
5. *A strong sense of ethics* (which includes an awareness of ethical codes and an acute awareness of upholding standards)
6. *Responsibility* (that is, accepting and knowing our own limitations).

Farrell and Gray (1992) give an example of this in a nursing context, such as anticipating the patient's need for a drink, staying close to a distressed patient or giving to a particular patient who is in need of more time. They point out that the wish to help others and to satisfy other people's needs is also fulfilling the practitioner's own personal and internal needs for self-esteem, social acceptance or being wanted.

Farrell and Gray also make a number of suggestions on how to respond in a therapeutic way to aggression in an attempt to avoid escalation. They argue that it is important to be supportive, to avoid defensiveness and to try to consider the feelings and thoughts of the aggressor and develop the skills of empathy. This involves careful, clear listening, tuning in to what the person may actually be saying underneath the words he or she uses (Farrell and Gray 1992). This is a very difficult skill, especially when confronted with anger or overt hostility, and can only be achieved with much practice. It is often difficult for practitioners to disengage from feelings of hurt and fear, and it is quite natural to withdraw or to become angry in response, which can, as will be discussed later, escalate the problem.

It is important that practitioners avoid situations in which the other person fears loss of face through backing down; where it is clear that there is a power struggle in progress, it is often more sensible to back down. Trying to recognise when this is happening is very important. It is clear that facile reassurances can make a situation far worse and, when in doubt, it is better to say nothing or say very little.

Wondrak (1989) has adapted five techniques in assertiveness training, first described by Smith (1975) as a possible way of enabling student nurses to deal more effectively with verbal abuse. The techniques are introduced in a workshop, and are fairly simple to use and understand, although they need to be practised in order to be used effectively. These will now be considered.

Five techniques for dealing with verbal abuse

The techniques consist of five main areas that can be adapted into a repertoire of skills:

1. Side-stepping
2. Self-disclosure
3. Partial agreement
4. Gentle confrontation
5. Being specific.

It is important to realise that the techniques are not a comprehensive way of dealing with all verbal attacks. The situation is usually a spontaneous one, confronting the practitioner unexpectedly and leaving, as discussed above, fear and apprehension, which often creates a blank. The techniques are, therefore, preferred as a way of raising consciousness and can be viewed in terms of preparing for the eventuality of a verbal attack; given the literature discussed earlier, the chances of the latter are fairly high. Again, the success of the situation depends on the context in which the incident is occurring. It will be important to consider the needs of the client, the situation in which it occurs, the disorder or condition affecting the individual and also the practitioner's feeling of confidence or ability to deal with the situation.

Side-stepping

The term 'side-stepping' seems to imply that the practitioner, when confronted, moves to one side as if avoiding possible confrontation; this is a useful analogy for the technique. It is a psychological technique whereby the individual responds totally non-defensively or non-aggressively and is very useful for dealing with spontaneous outbursts. Its basic function is to enable the practitioner to indicate what has been heard without becoming 'hooked' by what is being said.

Anxiety on behalf of the staff can often lead to over-control, which may make matters worse (Lowe 1992). The *intention* is to de-escalate threat and neutralise any possibility of the situation developing further. Side-stepping enables the individual to acknowledge the response while continuing to maintain self-esteem.

For example, in an encounter with a client who becomes angry and who may turn round suddenly and say 'Call yourself a nurse, you are b***** useless', a nurse can respond without trying to escalate the situation, without trying to argue back or justify his or her own usefulness, and simply reply, 'Yes, I agree, I have got a lot to learn.'

This can often help by taking the 'wind out of the client's sails' and immediately creates a surprise that wrongfoots the assailant. Care has to be taken that it is not repeated too often; there is nothing worse than trying to remain neutral when another is wanting an argument! However, it is important as a technique that can be used verbally, as well as non-verbally in the sense that side-stepping provides an attempt to step out of trouble.

It is important to be aware of the proximity of the person, and practitioners should check that they are in a position where they could retreat fairly quickly, not being backed into a wall or corner. This should become an important consideration at *all* times, especially where it is known that a client may be angry or may be behaving aggressively, or where there may be a history of aggression. It is surprising how often incidents occur that could have been avoided had the practitioner thought a bit more carefully about his or her positioning. Take the following story of a psychologist who walked into a room ahead of a client who had a history of violence. The client walked in behind, locked the door and put the catch down. When the psychologist enquired what he was doing, the response was, 'I am locking the door and then I am going to b***** kill you.' Such incidents help to clarify our thinking about the care we need to take in a very serious way when entering environments or situations from which it is difficult to escape; thus the skills of awareness and anticipation have to be developed at all times in the proximity of clients who are aggressive. In the story above, the psychologist was, fortunately, able to redeem the situation and calm the client down.

Self-disclosure

Used sensibly, this can often help the practitioner by reducing the anxiety of entering into an argument or discussion with someone who is angry or verbally aggressive. Nurses are often trapped by the 'professional image' they retain in order to deal with situations that may simply need honest and genuine responses. For example, the nurse may find it useful to tell the protagonist that he or she has been frightened or hurt by what has been said, or by disclosing simple statements such as 'I feel nervous when...' or 'I feel frightened when...' rather than drawing on false courage in an attempt to project a firm image of the nurse being in control. It is often the authoritarian stance, or the idea of being firmly in control, that can communicate non-verbally to a protagonist a clear threat, thus escalating the situation.

Partial agreement

This is a powerful technique that is used for dealing with hostile criticism from others by a simple technique of only agreeing with part of a criticism if it is appropriate. The important aspect is to accept what is said without arguing. For example, the best way to illustrate this technique is to give an example of a client being very critical of how a nurse looks. The situation may be such that the clients says:

I don't like the way you look, I hate the way you look, just look at all your clothes, you look a b***** mess!

The nurse may then say:

> Yes, you may be right there, these clothes don't go together and I dressed in a bit of a hurry this morning but they are comfortable, they are very comfortable.

This technique is to respond to criticism less defensively, listening to part of what is being said and agreeing to the bits that may be easier to accept. However, the nurse is also trying to assert some control by affirming his or her own position but not in an angry or aggressive way. This method seeks to treat the criticism by not validating what has been said or reacting to it as a serious accusation.

Gentle confrontation

This technique is possible once the client has become more amenable or is calming down. It follows on from 'partial agreement' and helps to encourage criticism in an attempt to focus not on the anger but on the substance – the reasons behind the hostility or anger. It can help to expose manipulation and constructively attempt to redirect the criticism. Following on from the previous example, the following extract may help to clarify this.

Client: You may like the effect and you may think you look comfortable, but I think you look stupid.

Nurse: I am not deliberately trying to dress to upset you but I can't help noticing that you do seem very upset about the way I look, and my dress seems to upset you more than it does me. Is there something else that is upsetting you today?

Thus the confrontation, switching from soaking up and agreeing with too much of what is being said, redirects a focus back to the protagonist in a fairly calm and gentle way.

Being specific

The final technique is often one that is very difficult to perform in stressful situations. However, with practice, it can be helpful. It is important to decide what it is you want to say or feel, and say it as clearly as possible, avoiding unnecessary padding. It is important to keep the statement simple and brief as it is then much more likely to be heard. This is more easily said than done, but with concentration and practice, it can be developed as a skill.

Debriefing

Whenever individuals have been involved in a situation in which they have been verbally abused or indeed on the receiving end of anger in any way, it is important that the individual *debriefs* the situation thoroughly with a colleague, mentor or supervisor. The process of debriefing simply means that the situation is related and described, and the context in which the situation arose is reconsidered, as are the events leading up to the incident itself. It is also very important for the individual to talk through the feelings that are left. Debriefing takes the form of the ability not only to reflect on what has happened, but also to look more critically at what was good about the way in which the incident was managed and perhaps what was not so good. Here again, no clear feedback is given following real incidents, and it is important to develop a clear structure in these discussions in which effective feedback can be offered.

Farrell and Gray (1992) offer some practical advice on giving feedback and suggest that individuals should avoid general statements and concentrate on focusing very specifically upon what occurred. It is important not to be detrimental and to give advice, but to remember that criticism may be interpreted in a painful way. It is important that adequate time and space are provided without too many interruptions. What is helpful after the event is a balanced view of what happened and to make time to arrange further meetings should it be necessary to revisit and re-reflect on the situation as a means of optimising learning (Farrell and Gray 1992).

After the event, particularly if the verbal abuse was very unpleasant, it is important to recognise that an individual may experience an acute reaction very similar to *post-traumatic stress disorder*, which is usually temporary but can sometimes continue unless it is dealt with through very effective support and debriefing. This condition is normally characterised by patterns of reactions that include re-experiencing the situation in an intrusive way, either in thoughts, dreams or nightmares; the individual may sometimes complain of a certain feeling that the incident is likely to happen again (Davidson-Neilson and Leick 1991).

'Avoidance behaviour' may also occur whereby the individual avoids all similar situations or environments, becomes restless and experiences sleeping and concentration difficulties. These reactions are normally fairly mild, and the anxiety disappears by itself in the course of a few weeks. However, such symptoms can continue in a way that shows the person is still affected by the experience, and in such instances it is important that this is recognised (Davidson-Nielson and Leick 1991). From the results of studies such as those of Cox (1987) cited above, indicating the reported high turnover of staff, it seems clear that there are significant traumatic affects of exposure to verbal abuse over a period of time. It, therefore, becomes important that techniques such as those described in this chapter are understood and practised, that consciousness is raised on this neglected area of violence and aggression, and that research continues to develop more effective and therapeutic ways of dealing with challenging behaviour.

References

Berkowitz L. (1962) *Aggression: A Social Psychological Analysis*, New York, McGraw-Hill.
Bernstein H.A. (1981) Survey of threats and assaults directed to psychotherapists, *American Journal of Psychotherapy*, **35**: 542–9.
Brammer L.M. (1979) *The Helping Relationship: Process and Skills*, 2nd edn, New Jersey, Prentice-Hall.
Buss A.H. (1961) *The Psychology of Aggression*, New York, John Wiley & Sons.
Caminski E.P., Whaley A.B., Whaley M.A. and Flaster M.L. (1984) *In Defense of a Dynamic Definition of Aggression*, Paper presented at the Annual Convention of the Speech Communication Association, Chicago.
Chitty K.K. and Maynard C.K. (1986) Managing manipulation, *Journal of Psycho-social Nursing*, **24**(6): 9–13.
Cox H.C. (1987) Verbal abuse in nursing: a report of a study, *Nursing Management*, **18**(11): 47–50.
Cox H.C. (1991) Verbal abuse nationwide, part 1: Oppressed group behaviour, *Nursing Management*, **22**(2): 32–5.
Curtin L. (1980) Sticks, stones and broken bones, *Supervisor Nurse*, **5** (December): editorial.
Davidson-Nielson M. and Leick N. (1991) *Healing Pain Attachment; Loss and Grief Therapy*, London, Routledge,
Duldt B.W. (1981) Anger: an alienating communication hazard for nurses, *Nursing Outlook*, November: 640–4.
Duldt B.W. (1982) Helping nurses to deal with the anger–dismay syndrome, *Nursing Outlook*, March: 168–74.
Farrell G.A. and Gray C. (1992) *Aggression: A Nurse's Guide to Therapeutic Management*, Scutari Press, London.

Fisher K. (1985) Charges catch clinicians in cycle of shame: slip ups, *APA Monitor*, May: 6–7.

Gordon I.T. and Green C.P. (1981) The impact of sexual stereotyping on health care: a nursing education workshop, *Journal of Nursing Education*, 20(4): 9.

Health and Safety Commission (1987) *Violence in the Health Service*, London, HMSO.

Infante D.A. (1987) Aggressiveness. In McCroskey J.C. and Daly J.A. (eds) *Personal and Interpersonal Communication*, 6: 157–19, Newbury Park, CA, Sage.

Infante D.A. and Rancer A.S. (1982) A conceptualisation and measure of argumentativeness, *Journal of Personality Assessment*, 46: 72–80.

Kalogerakis M.G. (1971) The assaultive psychiatric patient, *Psychiatric Quarterly*, 44: 3372–81.

Kohnke M.F. (1981) Nurse abuse – nurse abusers, *Nursing and Health Care*, May: 256–60.

Lion J.R. and Reid W.H. (1983) *Assaults within Psychiatric Facilities*, New York, Grune & Stratton.

Lowe T. (1992) Characteristics of effective nursing interventions in the management of challenging behaviour, *Journal of Advanced Nursing*, 17: 1226–32.

McCroskey J.C. and Daly J.A. (1987) *Personality and Interpersonal Communication*, Newbury Park, CA, Sage.

Reakes J.T. (1981) Nurse abuse, *Texas Nursing*, October: 8–11.

Remland M. (1982) The implicit adhominem fallacy: non verbal displays of status in argumentative discourse, *Journal of the American Forensic Association*, 19: 79–86.

Sanford K.D. (1985) How to cope with nurse abuse, *Nursing Life*, September/October: 52–5.

Self P.R. and Vieu J.J. (1980) Four steps for helping a patient alleviate anger, *Nursing* (US), 10(12): 66.

Smith M. (1975) *When I Say No I Feel Guilty*, London, Bantam Books.

Tedeschi J.T. (1983) Social influence theory and aggression. In Green R.G. and Donnerstein E.I. (eds) *Aggression: Theoretical and Empirical Reviews* 1: 135–62, New York, Academic Press.

Torres G. (1981) Nursing education administrator: accountable, vulnerable and depressed, *Advances in Nursing Science*, 3(3): 115.

Tyron G.S. (1986) Abuse of therapists by patients: a national survey, *Professional Psychology Research and Practice*, 17(4): 357–63.

Whitman R.M., Armao B.B. and Dent O.B. (1976) Assaults on the therapist, *American Journal of Psychiatry*, 133: 426–9.

Wondrak R. (1989) Dealing with verbal abuse, *Nurse Education Today*, 9: 276–80.

6

DE-ESCALATION IN THE MANAGEMENT OF AGGRESSION AND VIOLENCE: TOWARDS EVIDENCE-BASED PRACTICE

Brodie Paterson and David Leadbetter

Total organisational response

In its original usage, the concept of de-escalation is simple. It implies the existence of a set of verbal and non-verbal skills which, if used selectively and appropriately, may reduce the level of an aggressor's hostility by calming anger and lowering arousal. As a consequence of doing so, it is suggested that the associated risk of assaultive behaviour in a crisis situation will decrease (Turnbull *et al.* 1990, Stevenson 1991). The term 'de-escalation' is to be preferred to alternatives sometimes employed, such as 'talkdown' or 'defusing' because it more accurately describes the process involved. The skills employed are neither intuitive nor instinctual and do not always result from experience. They require skilled teaching and supervised practice to achieve competence in their application (Paterson 1994).

This chapter will first review the role of the organisation in de-escalation before exploring the underlying theory and practice of de-escalation through reference to two alternative attempts to model the process.

It has been suggested that the concept of de-escalation should be applied in a broader sense to encompass the role of the organisation, including its culture, organisation, policies and procedures (Leadbetter and Paterson 1995).

This perspective argues that organisations have a firmly identified responsibility in legislation to be proactive in identifying and reducing the risk to which staff are exposed from aggression and violence (Stark and Kidd 1995). This process of risk assessment and reduction is seen as an essential element of de-escalation in the prevention and pre-emption of incidents (Greaves 1994).

If, for example, the issue of perceived excessive waiting time were identified as one factor involved in the triggering of aggressive incidents in an accident and emergency department, individuals within that department would have a responsibility to bring that to the attention of the organisation. The organisation would have a responsibility both to act to identify the risks its workers faced (that is, it is no longer a defence for it to say that it did not know there was a problem) and to respond to concerns identified by whatever means to try to reduce waiting time. The management of aggressive and violent behaviour must be seen within a context in which both the individual and the organisation, working in partnership, have an active role in taking steps to reduce the likelihood of violence and in forming and maintaining social norms against violence. Viewing de-escalation solely as the responsibility of the individual practitioner is, therefore, inappropriate. The practice of de-escalation by teams and individuals forms only one part of the co-ordinated effort that is a necessary prerequisite of effective action at the level of the organisation. The underlying idea is of a 'total organisational response' (Cox and Cox 1993), encompassing issues such as building design, service culture and values (Fein *et al.* 1981), operational policies, procedures and working practices (Rice *et al.* 1989), core staff skills and training, complementing the actions of individual practitioners.

The remit of de-escalation will vary depending on the context within which it is practised. De-escalation in some care settings may form only one element within a treatment package that should incorporate (La Vigna and Donnellan 1986):

- *Environmental management*: the identification and modification of triggers and setting conditions for violence
- *Positive programming*: increasing client adaptive engagement
- *Focused intervention*: targeting underlying skills or values deficits and eliminating contingencies that may be maintaining behaviour
- *Reactive strategies*: de-escalation and physical restraint.

Core values and skills

Lowe (1992), Farrell and Grey (1992) and Leadbetter and Paterson (1995) argue that good practice in the management of aggressive behaviour is built upon a core base of values and skills that underlie practice. These include:

■ *Consistent respect for the intrinsic value and dignity of the individual*
All nursing practice is based upon the premise that individuals are deserving of respect and dignity no matter what their circumstances or behaviour. All therapeutic work starts from the acceptance of this principle.

■ *An empathic non-judgemental approach*
Empathy is the ability accurately to recognise another's perspective and feelings, and to communicate to the person an understanding of his or her perspective. In potentially aggressive situations, this involves the ability to recognise the emotion being experienced by the client and to try to understand the reasons behind it, both immediately and in the longer term.

■ *Honesty*
The concept of genuineness is common to several therapeutic approaches but can be summarised using an information technology analogy as 'what you see is what you get'. It is associated with the concept of integrity, which, while complex, involves notions of consistency, justice and concern for the welfare of others.

■ *Self-awareness*
Self-awareness is a fundamental skill in nursing with regard to an in-depth knowledge of who we are in terms of our values and attitudes. It is also crucial to understand and recognise the impact of our behaviour on others and vice versa in our interactions with others.

■ *Communication skills*
The ability to communicate clearly, unambiguously and effectively is central to good practice in any context. De-escalation requires exceptionally close attention to the process of communication.

Consensus and de-escalation – an impossible task?

A difficult problem facing a reader new to this area who is looking for guidance for practice is the lack of consensus on how de-escalation is to be carried out. This lack of consensus is reflected in the conflicting approaches to developing theoretical models of de-escalation. There is evidently no standardised approach to the process of de-escalation, and one of the problems facing the reviewer is that the various approaches may offer differing and even mutually contradictory advice (Breakwell 1989). The conflicting advice seems to stem from the complexity of the issues of aggression and violence, the wide variety of theoretical explanations offered and a continuing lack of systematic research in the area of de-escalation to evaluate the effectiveness of competing models empirically (Paterson *et al.* 1992).

In the literature on de-escalation, a variety of differing approaches to determining the constituents of the process are evident. A number of authors do not adopt or identify any particular theoretical framework to underpin their approach. Advice on practice is given within a theoretical framework, which can be criticised for failing to provide a coherent or cogent basis for the approach advocated. A range of models has been used in a variety of different ways to provide the basis for the development of models of de-escalation, including cognitive psychology (Turnbull *et al.* 1990) and transactional analysis (Farrell and Gray 1992) among others. In addition, a variety of models have been proposed, which can be broadly categorised as 'eclectic', that attempt to integrate insights from a variety of perspectives (Blair 1991).

De-escalation and theoretical explanations of violence

Any theory of de-escalation must have an implicit or explicit view on why aggression and violence occur. The aetiology of aggression is inordinately complex, but the underlying perspective taken in this chapter on why aggression occurs is ecological (Leadbetter and Paterson 1995), viewing aggression as being multiply determined (Siann 1985). It sees aggression as arising as a consequence of the interactions within individuals in terms of their physiological make-up, personality, learning history, culture, predisposing interactional style (Leadbetter and Paterson 1995) and cognitive appraisal of the situations and events they have experienced and are experiencing, including their interactions with others (Steadman 1982) (Figure 6.1).

If the compelling logic that aggression is multiply determined is accepted, any model of de-escalation must attempt to identify which factors may be available and amenable to manipulation or elimination in a way that reduces the risk of violence occurring. It is acknowledged that some factors that may be significant contributory elements in some situations, such as those where the client has an organic brain disorder or is suffering from drug intoxication, may not be immediately available for manipulation. However, the idea is to try to work with what is available in the short term while working towards a constructive resolution in the longer term.

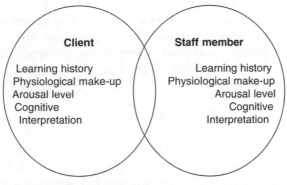

Figure 6.1 An interactional model of violence

The multimodal approach

This chapter will adopt what will be termed a 'multimodal' approach. The basic premise is that if we recognise that a behaviour is affected by a variety of factors, attempts to change a behaviour will be more successful if as many of the possible variables affecting the behaviour can be recognised and changed. The basis of this approach is the attempt to create a coherent theoretical framework to explain why particular de-escalation strategies are advocated and how these techniques should be applied through an analysis and synthesis of relevant theory and research.

Incident modelling

A useful and relatively simple conceptual model of the necessary ingredients for a violent incident is provided by Bailey (1977). He proposes that violent incidents need four elements:

a trigger *a high level of arousal*
a target *a weapon*

The removal of any element will reduce the risk of violence. The approach has similarities to that adopted in fire prevention, which may be familiar to some readers. Three ingredients are necessary for a fire: fuel, heat and oxygen. Remove the presence of any one element and you can prevent (or put out) a fire.

Arousal

Arousal is an innate response to anxiety-provoking situations with physiological features sometimes referred to as the fight or flight reaction. Arousal in itself is not intrinsically associated with anger and hostility, but it appears to be strongly linked to aggression and violence (Averill 1982) as a consequence of its effect on the cognitions, emotion and behaviour of the individual and the instinctual desire to reduce high levels of arousal (Breakwell and Rowett 1989). Novaco (1976) observed that anger as a form of arousal is a consequence of an interpretation of a event or incident as being provocative. His perspective views emotion largely as a consequence of an internal mental process involving an interaction between an 'event' which may be overt or covert, the interpretation of that event for meaning, which will influence and be influenced by an emotional response and in turn influence behaviour which being overt or covert may form a subsequent event (see Figure 6.2).

Novaco (1975, 1976) argues that events provoke anger only in the way in which the individual interprets them. All individuals have their own unique way of interpreting the world around them, which will determine their reaction to an event (Novaco 1977). Of note is the observation that the interaction between arousal and anger may be invidious in that, while under stress and thus aroused, one may be more likely to make negative attributions with regard to the actions of or intent of others and thus likely continually to trigger thoughts maintaining and producing anger and high arousal (Mueller 1983).

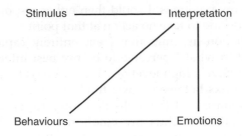

Figure 6.2   Interaction between events interpretation and arousal

A variety of examples can be used to illustrate this process. If, for example, someone spills my drink in a public house, my reaction to the event is affected by a variety of factors. Some of these are 'external' that is, they are going on in the world around me. Some, however, are 'internal' – they are my interpretation of the events. In considering external factors, we might note whether the person who spilled our drink was bumped by someone else, whether the pub was extremely busy, whether the person was showing signs of being drunk and whether it was the local 'hard man' with a reputation for violence. We would also conduct an internal appraisal of the event. Was the spilling of the drink deliberate or accidental? (Note that this attribution of intent is crucially a product of an internal appraisal. It is what I think he did rather than what he actually did that will influence my reaction.) Has the person's apology and offer to replace the drink done enough to restore my potential loss of face among my peers? Will I lose status if I do not respond to this incident aggressively? What do my peer group expect me to do in a situation like this? Does the person need to be 'taught a lesson' to ensure that he does not do it again? What will the consequences be for me if I become aggressive?

My interpretation of the events will determine my emotional response. If I believe that the spilled drink represents a deliberate slight, I would consider that the person had insulted me (perhaps in front of my peer group). My thoughts might revolve around themes such as: How dare that b****** do that to me; who the hell does he think he is? Such self-statements act to trigger an emotional response that has a physiological component that, over time, I have learned represents my anger and gives me a rationale for being aggressive. Depending on my ability to exercise control over my thought process and therefore my emotions, I could then either respond verbally or physically, or decide to take no action at that point.

This explanation assumes that I am entirely capable of acting rationally and in what I perceive to be my best interest. It further assumes that I have a high level of self-awareness that allows me to recognise the links between how I think, what I am thinking, my emotional response and the skills necessary to try to change my train of thoughts and thus my emotional state. The process is similar to that of changing a tape recording. If the recording that is playing is provoking anger and I do not want to be angry at this time, I can try to replace it with something more suitable. The process can, in principle, be described in very simple terms, and to some extent the skills are intuitively used by most people.

Learning to use 'self-talk' as a means of controlling our behaviour is, however, a cognitive skill, which in the course of normal development initially occurs from about 3 years onwards. In practice, some people may not have learned these skills or may be unable to use them for a variety of reasons, either permanently as the result of a brain injury, or temporarily as a result of drug intoxication.

If a client verbally abuses me, and what we define as verbal abuse depends on who we are, or attempts to assault me, my initial reaction might then be to think, 'Why me, what have I done to deserve this? I'm here trying to help and this person is insulting/assaulting me; why should I bother?' This vein of thought will very quickly produce anger in terms of the feelings of arousal. It is, however, inappropriate because I cannot necessarily leave the person or refuse to continue his or her treatment, and it may be counterproductive to allow myself to become angry because, depending on the degree of arousal associated with my anger, my judgement may become impaired. If I interpret another's actions as provocative, I have a rationale for my subsequent behaviour. It is important to recognise that aggressors may believe that their actions are justified by the circumstances and that they had no choice but to act (Toch 1969).

A significant potential weakness of Bailey's model relates to his view that arousal is a necessary ingredient for violence. A conventional theoretical distinction divides aggression into two categories: 'hostile' and 'instrumental'. Hostile aggression is that associated with high arousal and anger. In contrast, in instrumental aggression, anger and arousal are absent, and the aggression is displayed in order to achieve a specific goal (Weisfeld 1994). In individual instances, the relative motivation behind aggression will vary, either or both facets of aggression being present to a greater or lesser degree.

In an instance of domestic violence, a man may be angry at his partner and at the same time be aware that to use violence will enable him to assert his dominance in the relationship (Berkowitz 1993). Where someone chooses to rob a bank, the aggression he or she displays can be both instrumental and hostile. The instrumental aggression stems from what may be a considered decision involving detailed planning to use force or the threat of force to rob a bank. The hostile aggression is likely to occur as a consequence of the anxiety-provoking experience of the actual robbery.

Triggers

Certain circumstances and interpretations of circumstances may act as triggers that act to move arousal levels upwards from some notional baseline towards a crisis, and one crucial element of de-escalation is to attempt to avoid triggering behaviours. The concept of a trigger is best explained with reference to Kaplan and Wheeler's (1983) 'assault cycle'. They describe incidents as having five phases:

1. The triggering phase
2. The escalation phase
3. The crisis phase
4. The recovery phase
5. The depression phase.

Incidents can be triggered by a range of circumstances. Fixing limits on client and patient behaviour where such behaviour has consequences for the client or others can sometimes be a necessary part of nurses' and other health professionals' role. It must be handled carefully and sympathetically, however, for the client or patient's anger and hostility at the situation or the system can easily be displaced towards the available target of the staff (Breakwell and Rowett 1989). It must also be done consistently to avoid the client interpreting the application of limits as having personal overtones, as in 'I was allowed to do this yesterday by Joe Bloggs. If I am not allowed to do this today it must be because you do not like me or are picking on me' (Madden 1977). Training in non-confrontational methods of limit-setting such as contingency contracting can contribute to a reduction the incidence of violence (Infantino and Musingo 1985).

Triggers for situations may be non-verbal in that angry and aroused people have an increased need for personal space. Nurses can, therefore, provoke incidents by not respecting this need for increased distance (Negley and Manley 1990, Blair 1991) or by unwittingly adopting a confrontational stance or posture. Standing directly in front of a client who is angry is advised against by Turnbull *et al.* (1990) and Leadbetter and Paterson (1995). The staff member should use a stance placing him or herself at an angle of approximately 45 degrees to the client, whether standing or sitting (Davies 1989). The posture adopted in conjunction with this stance should show interest and concern but not aggression, with the hands held palms open in view of the client out of any pockets and neither placed on the hips nor folded, which may be seen as aggressive (Mehrabian 1969). The stance and posture described demonstrates minimum threat to the client but is not submissive (Mehrabian 1972). In addition, from a practical perspective, it readily forms the basis for a 'defensive' posture should violence occur (Leadbetter and Paterson 1995). If the client is approached, this should be done slowly and carefully from a direction from which the nurse's advance can clearly be seen by the client to minimise any potential threat (Burrow 1994).

The use of touch with someone who is highly aroused requires extreme care (Barlow 1989, Conlon *et al.* 1995). Nurses and other health care professionals may be allowed to violate the taboos regarding touch in our society, but this must always be done in ways that respect the dignity and individuality of clients. In a situation where a client is angry, it should either be avoided altogether (MacDonnell *et al.* 1994) or done slowly and preferably with the client's explicit permission in order to avoid misinterpretation (Gertz 1980).

Close attention should also be paid to eye contact, which should attempt to remain akin to that occurring in normal conversation. Prolonged direct eye contact in a situation where a client is highly aroused is generally to be avoided because it may be interpreted provocatively, while the avoidance of contact may be viewed as being submissive or fearful (Rice *et al.* 1990, Turnbull *et al.* 1990).

The issue of race, ethnicity and culture, and its relationship to non-verbal communication, is extremely complex and outside the scope of discussion of this chapter. It is important to note, however, that as language and dialect vary between cultures, so does non-verbal communication. Caution and sensitivity must, therefore, be exercised in applying the advice given in different contexts where the participants have differing cultural backgrounds (Morton 1986).

Other triggers may be verbal, where a certain phrase associated with something emotive for the client provokes anger (Breakwell 1989). Many readers will understand from experience of childhood or parenthood the way in which siblings can induce anger by knowing exactly 'which buttons to push'. In practice, knowledge and experience with a client can allow staff to identify and avoid certain triggers, but this is more difficult with unfamiliar clients. Accordingly, close attention to the content of verbal communication and the client's reaction, both verbally and non-verbally, is a priority both during incidents and in post-incident analysis in order to identify and avoid inadvertently triggering anger. These triggers can, however, serve as a focus for exploration after crisis.

Weapon

A weapon in Bailey's model is something that can be used to hurt someone. This includes the client's fists, feet, head and teeth as well as what may be more generally perceived as a weapon. It is thus impossible to restrict clients' access to any kind of weapon. Obvious advice in areas of high risk is to keep sharp objects secured in areas away from unsupervised access by clients and to establish and use security procedures to try to prevent the introduction or construction of weapons (Rice *et al.* 1989).

Target

In an aggressive incident, the role of the 'target' (which can be a staff member, fellow client or aggressors themselves) is to provide a recipient for the aggression of the assailant. A wide variety of factors may affect the likelihood of an individual staff member being a victim of assault, including their gender relative to the assailant (Stark *et al.* 1995), their attitude (Morrison 1990) and their exposure in terms of time spent directly interacting with clients. The preceding discussion has strongly argued that an additional intervening variable is their behaviour.

In attempting to ensure that the staff member is not seen as a legitimate target, a number of strategies have been identified.

Clear guidelines that any assault on a member of staff will result in police involvement may act to deter assault by increasing the potential tariff for violence. Where the primary motivation for assault is instrumental, this may have the effect of causing the person to reconsider the consequences of his or her behaviour (Tardiff 1989). If the client's anger is a consequence of a perceived failure of the system or a conflict with the rules of the system, it can be helpful if members of staff can act to personalise themselves so that they are seen as individuals rather than faceless representatives of the system, against whom the aggressor may have a grievance. If the system or an individual has been at fault, a prompt apology is appropriate.

A pre-existing relationship with the client should be of value in two ways. First, if a therapeutic relationship has been developed, the trust that forms part of that relationship can be used as a means of displacing the aggression on to a more appropriate means of complaining. Second, previous knowledge of the client may give some clues to the strategies most likely to work with any given individual, although it is important to note that what worked before with an individual will not necessarily work again.

Some staff may unwittingly act provocatively in attempting to de-escalate incidents. Traditionally, consistent advice has been given that staff should remain calm (Breakwell 1989) and 'model calmness' in their interactions with highly aroused people (MacDonnell *et al.* 1994). This advice remains appropriate but requires some elaboration as there can be an unwitting problem in modelling calmness. Michael Argyle (1983) describes a phenomenon of interpersonal communication that he calls 'mirroring'. It is a convention in which the emotional level in terms of arousal evident in speech is generally to some extent mirrored in the responses of the listener. If I came into work and I was extremely happy because something wonderful had happened in my life (like Glasgow Celtic winning the European cup again – please allow me a moment of authorial fantasy), then if your response to my apparent delight was extremely cool, I would be both disappointed and disconcerted because you had failed to observe the appropriate convention. (You could of course be a Glasgow Rangers fan, in which case your coolness might be understandable!) In a more serious vein, if I am extremely angry and you respond to me with absolute calm, I might perceive your response as patronising and non-empathetic or as a form of passive aggression. I might even, because you have failed to react in the way in which I expected, raise the level of my aggression from verbal to physical in order to provoke the desired response.

Davies (1989) argues that applying the principle of mirroring to de-escalation requires that we consider 'mood-matching', in which we overtly and deliberately display signs of increased arousal such as raising the pitch and volume of our voice in response to high arousal in the client. The idea is to move towards matching the level of overt arousal and then to model a gradual reduction in arousal. The convention of mirroring should, if operating, then influence the client to respond by reducing his or her overt arousal. If, for example, a client were shouting loudly and not responding to attempts to calmly intervene, it would be appropriate to test out raising the volume of the voice momentarily to gain their attention (Breakwell 1989).

Somewhat confusingly, despite Davies' use of the term 'mood-matching', the intention is clearly *not* for the staff member to match the mood or emotion of the clients but to display signs of *apparently* heightened arousal, such as raising the volume of the voice momentarily (Turnbull *et al.* 1990). In attempting to de-escalate a situation, displaying anger is very unlikely to lead to a constructive resolution of a situation. MacDonnell *et al.* (1994) have suggested that the distinction between emotional content and arousal level may be difficult for staff to grasp and thus potentially dangerous if the aggressor perceives an individual as matching the emotional content as well as the arousal level. This criticism is not supported by the research of Paterson *et al.* (1992), who found it possible to teach care staff to use mood-matching appropriately and effectively as part of a programme of training in de-escalation.

In certain circumstances, staff may accidentally contribute to the aggressive content of a situation by what they say. The role of certain expressions as being provocative is clear, and, for example, to insult someone is understandably to risk triggering aggression. On occasions, however, staff may unintentionally provoke aggression through the indiscriminate use of phrases such as 'Calm down', 'Don't be silly', 'I can understand how you feel' or 'I can see you're angry.' The problem with such phrases is not the intention behind them, which may be laudable, but the danger that the client may perceive them as indicative of a patronising attitude (Turnbull *et al.* 1990).

A final potential element to note with regard to decreasing the potential for victimisation is to consider the role of the audience. The presence of an audience to an aggressive incident will have an effect that can be positive or negative with regard to de-escalation. The audience may be available for manipulation by both the aggressor and the staff member, and its effect should be judged and acted upon.

If an audience is perceived as having a negative effect (for example, it may be more difficult for an aggressor to compromise in front of his or her peers), attempts should be made to remove the individual from the audience or vice versa (Turnbull *et al.* 1990). In doing so, the risk involved in interviewing a potentially aggressive individual on one's own should be reviewed and the potential for escape or readily available assistance considered. If a situation involving the presence of an audience deteriorates, it may be necessary to make a direct request to an individual member of the audience for assistance in overcoming the diffusion of responsibility that can occur within groups (Breakwell 1989).

Judgements and decisions

Aggressive situations can be perceived as a state of flux. The behaviour of staff in attempting de-escalation is one in which they continually make judgements during the process, decide and implement their response, and monitor and evaluate the impact of their actions and what else is happening in the environment on the aggressor. The aim of the process is to work towards the constructive resolution of a crisis by testing out particular strategies (Example 6.1).

Example 6.1

It is early Saturday morning in a psychiatric intensive care unit. Louise, a 34-year-old client, has shown signs of being increasingly distraught, pacing up and down in the sitting room and talking to herself quite loudly. She has angrily resisted earlier discreet attempts to divert her to her room and prompts to engage in self-management strategies for her auditory hallucinations, which she appears to be experiencing. She has also refused offers of medication. Suddenly, she begins to accuse a fellow patient of laughing at her and starts threatening to 'sort her out'. The other client responds angrily, threatening to assault her. Both clients have been violent in the past.

Issues for judgement here include:

■ Are the audience (the other clients/staff) liable to play a constructive role in this situation or not?
■ Is Louise's aggression primarily instrumental or hostile?

- What is the level of her arousal, and is it going up or down?
- Is the source of her aggression immediately identifiable and amenable to resolution?
- What potential risk do Louise and the other client pose to each other's welfare?
- Would another member of staff who has a better relationship with Louise increase the likelihood of a successful resolution of this situation?

From such judgements flow decisions in relation to:

- Should I try to separate these two clients, and how?
- Should I stay here where other staff members can discreetly observe, or invite Louise or the other client to come into the office to discuss this?
- Should I ask questions/give choices or be directive?
- Should I model calmness or mood-match?
- Should I inform Louise and the other client of the potential tariffs if they become violent?
- Should I move towards Louise or away, and how close should I get to her?
- Should I use touch or not?
- Should I ask another member of staff to talk to Louise?

There are no absolute right or wrong answers, although it is likely that calm intervention, perhaps discreetly placing staff members where they could get between both clients if necessary and trying to prompt one to leave temporarily, represents the first steps. Subsequent staff actions should be guided by the situation as it evolves. In a given incident, effective de-escalation could require the member of staff to use, for example, modelling calmness and mood-matching at different times in the same incident depending on the client's behaviour and response to the actions of staff. Practice is thus customised to suit the individual and the situation within a general framework, which may variously encompass the following:

triggers	*high level of arousal*
Set limits sensitively and consistently	Distract from the source of arousal by questioning/negotiating
Avoid direct prolonged eye contact	Provide face-saving alternatives that maintain the client's dignity

Attend to stance and posture
Avoid provocative phrases
Avoid crowding the individual
and give more space

Acknowledge the emotional content
of speech but avoid labelling
Give clear, specific, unambiguous,
concrete messages
Try to problem-solve; focus on
something that can be done

target
Personalise self
Manage the audience
Communicate the potential tariff
for assault
Model calmness or mood-
match depending on the situation
and response
Apologise; do not defend a bad
system
Do not make promises you or
other staff cannot keep (unless
it is to protect yourself from
immediate physical danger)

weapon
Manage the environment and workplace design
Discreetly remove potential
weapons during acute crisis

Stabilising flux

Leadbetter (1993) and Leadbetter and Paterson (1995) have suggested that a potential refinement of existing models of de-escalation can be achieved by considering Kaplan and Wheeler's (1983) assault cycle described earlier and determining where specific de-escalation strategies are applicable across the assault cycle. This model titled CALM (Crisis Aggression Limitation and Management) represents a stage-specific approach to the process of de-escalation, which starts before and ends after the incident itself. The model is attractive both theoretically and ideologically, but it may potentially depend on whether staff can reliably discern where a client is in the assault cycle, which is not yet established. It is presently subject to evaluative research.

The model is based on a series of underlying assumptions (Leadbetter and Trewartha 1996):

■ The factors that influence behaviour are liable to change in nature and relevance as the person's arousal level changes as a product of the influence of rising arousal on cognition.

■ The ability of the staff member to match his or her response to the overt and covert emotion of the client is central to the likelihood of a successful outcome.

■ The staff member's own emotional reaction and the sense of threat in the aggressor's behaviour are probably the best gauge of the aggressor's behaviour in the arousal cycle.

Behaviour in adults is usually under a significant degree of cognitive control, so we can appraise a situation, make a judgement, consider our response and act. In the initial stages of a confrontation, therefore, rational argument is a primary tool. Cognitive control will, however, rapidly decline as arousal increases and emotion moves to become the predominant influence on behaviour. Anecdotally, there are many examples of situations in which the victim conceded to the demands of the aggressor but was still assaulted, possibly because the aggressor's arousal ultimately overwhelmed their rational self-interest.

Pre-incident

■ Develop an understanding of policies and protocols.
■ Implement violent incident drills.
■ Develop staff support networks.
■ Promote open discussion and an exchange of information.
■ Conduct a risk assessment of units or services.
■ Identify and modify facilities and practices as appropriate.

Phase 1: The onset of arousal responding to increased anxiety

Dominant emotion: anxiety
Aim of intervention: calming.

Actions

■ Monitor the client's emotional state.
■ Identify and resolve immediate and underlying problems.
■ Aid the client to reduce anxiety.
■ Establish a rapport.

Strategies

- *Personalise.* Use names and previous relationships.
- *Paraphrase and summarise.* Repeat statements, checking for understanding.
- *Reflect feeling.* Comment on feelings and identify them: 'I appreciate that you are angry.'
- *Reassure.* Praise the client for expressing emotions: 'It's OK to be angry/upset' and so on.
- *Use open questions.* Encourage exploration of the problem/situation.
- *Use relaxation.* Encourage the client to use a relaxation strategy, for example, breathing exercises for panic or autogenic relaxation.
- *Involve or divert.* Redirect the client into available activities.
- *Planned ignoring.* Use this only as part of formal strategy where functional analysis indicates inappropriate attention-seeking and no possibility of escalation.
- *Use non-verbal skills.* Convey interest and empathy by adopting an open attentive posture.

Try to avoid:
- *Why questions.* These may prompt the person to rehearse reasons for his or her anxiety and/or invoke a defensive response, both of which could escalate the situation.
- *Closed questions.* Simple yes/no answers will not be terribly helpful.
- *Complicated questions.* These increase the likelihood of misunderstanding.
- *Conveying threat.* Avoid behaviour that might be interpreted as authoritarian or patronising.

Phase 2: Dealing with increasingly angry behaviour

Dominant emotion: anxiety/anger
Aim of intervention: calming and/or de-escalation.

This phase is essentially transitional, and the staff member must exercise judgement on the dominant emotion in the situation and be prepared to adjust his or her actions accordingly based on this perception. If anger is predominating and escalating, the required response is to move from a focus on assisting the client to a focus on risk reduction by de-escalation. This will require a conscious shift to the processes characteristic of phase 3.

Phase 3: Dealing with the onset of aggressive behaviour

Dominant emotion: anger
Aim of intervention: de-escalation.

Actions

■ Prevent further escalation.
■ Reduce emotional arousal.
■ Redirect and re-engage thinking away from the anger.

Strategies

■ *Encourage dialogue.* Keep the person talking (intervene if direction is negative).
■ *Use silence.* Allowing silence may also be helpful.
■ *Non-verbal aspects.* Give space. Attend to one's own and the client's posture, stance, facial expression and eye contact.
■ *Use arousal.* Use low arousal, a calm tone and a low but clear volume. Use mood-matching arousal with momentary shouting followed by a reduction in pitch and volume.
■ *Use distraction.* Distract the client by seeking detailed information by giving choices or by attempting to change the focus.
■ *Use limits.* For example, 'Once you stop shouting I will listen to you.'
■ *Negotiate.* Avoid unnecessary confrontation. Try to negotiate mutually acceptable outcomes. Work using the little-to-large principle (trying to gain small concessions first).
■ *Give direction.* 'Stop now.'
■ *Use disclosure.* Remind the aggressor that you are a person with a family and so on and not just a faceless representative of a 'system' against which he or she may have a grievance. Consider the disclosure of emotions, for example 'You're frightening me.'
■ *Consequences.* Inform the client of the consequences of the behaviour. 'It's our policy to involve the police if...'. Great care *must* be taken if this is done to avoid its being perceived as a threat.
■ *Use the audience.* If the contribution of an audience of other clients is unhelpful, try to separate the client from the audience as discreetly as possible. If you believe that they may be beneficial, try to counteract the 'bystander phenomenon' by making a direct appeal for support.

- *Use humour.* Apply this with caution and only if you can be reasonably sure that what you say will be perceived as funny by the client.

If the behaviour continues to escalate:
- *Summon help.* If possible, do this discreetly to avoid cueing violence. Prior arrangements for emergency situations should always be in place before rather than after a disaster.
- *Offer medication.* If prescribed.
- *Withdraw.* In some situations, discretion should take precedence over valour.
- *Remove weapons.* Remove objects with an obvious potential to be used as weapons. This must be done with great discretion to avoid providing a cue for violence.

Try to avoid:
- Counteraggression anger
- Postponement/displacement to other staff, for example 'You'll need to take that up with...'
- Making promises that you or others will not be able to keep
- Threats
- Touch
- Discussion/exploration of feelings
- Invasion of the client's space
- Unrealistic expectations
- Verbal expressions such as 'Calm down' or 'Don't be silly'.

Phase 4: Dealing with physically violent behaviour

Dominant emotion: hostility
Aim of intervention: to maintain the safety of staff and client(s) – escape and/or restraint.

Actions

- Ensure the safety of staff.
- Ensure the safety of client(s).
- Ensure the safety of bystanders.

Strategies

- Communication of unacceptability
- Escape

- Self-defence/breakaway techniques
- Restraint
- Medication
- Seclusion.

Try to avoid:
- Freezing
- Over-reacting, especially the use of excessive force
- Panic
- Actions based on a desire for retribution.

Phase 5: Dealing with aggression once the person is no longer physically violent

Dominant emotion: anger/anxiety
Aims of intervention: risk reduction, re-engagement.

Actions

These will vary depending on the context and location of the incident and the operational policy of the organisation concerned. Key tasks are to:

- Stop physical restraint as soon as possible compatible with maintaining continuing safety for staff and client(s). This should be done through a gradual relaxation of restraint accompanying reductions in the client's overtly threatening behaviour and level of arousal.
- Maintain supervision.
- Relieve staff and provide additional resources.
- Use medication if absolutely necessary.
- Obtain medical advice or first aid if necessary.
- Obtain *expert* advice on continuing management *early* if aggression is prolonged.
- Involve senior management or security staff.

Things to avoid:
- Re-igniting situation
- Retaliation
- An early discussion of consequences, which might be perceived by the person as being punitive. These may be less likely to be perceived as simply retaliation when the person is calm.

- Attempting to engage in complex problem-solving too early. This should be deferred to a time at which the person has calmed down.

Phase 6: Dealing with lessening but persistent arousal

Dominant emotion: anger
Aim of intervention: problem-solving.

Actions

- Minimise the perceived positive potential effects of the use of aggression.
- Resolve, where possible, any underlying problems that may have acted as a trigger for the incident.
- Identify alternative strategies for future use by the client in other situations.
- Support the legitimacy of the organisation's rules and expectations.

Strategies

- *Allow space*
  A cup of tea and/or a cigarette, for example, for both staff and client when the client's behaviour suggests a diminishing risk may provide a useful cooling-off period. Be aware, however, that adrenaline will continue to affect the client's arousal for approximately 90 minutes after an incident, and be careful, therefore, not to unwittingly trigger another incident during this period when the client's sensitivity may be heightened
- *Problem-solve*
  Attempt to identify triggers and overt and covert reasons for the incident. Problem-solve either indirectly by facilitating the person in exploring his or her perspective and any alternative interpretations or directly by giving advice and information on alternative strategies.

Try to avoid:
- Triggering another incident by prompting a rehearsal of the client's original reason for the anger
- Punitive approaches, either overtly or covertly
- Relaxing vigilance too early.

Phase 7: Helping an aggressor to learn from an incident

Dominant emotions: anxiety, contrition, exhaustion, focused anger
Aim of intervention: debriefing.

Actions

■ Promote adaptive learning.
■ Increase the client's insight into his or her behaviour.
■ Identify and practise alternative functional behaviours.
■ Re-engage the person in normal activities.

Strategies

■ *Debriefing*
A crisis can provide the individuals concerned with an opportunity for personal development and growth. In some instances, aggression is a consequence of the client's dysfunctional interpretation of events that has evoked anger and thus aggression. The person may lack the skills necessary either to manage positively the situation or the emotions it generates. For some clients, the motivation to change exists, and dysfunctional interpretations can be challenged and altered, and/or skills to deal with heightened arousal taught and learned (Neizo and Lanza 1984). This requires commitment on the part of both staff and the aggressor.

An aggressive incident, with the attendant passions it generates, constitutes both a problem and an opportunity. Unfortunately, in many situations, the positive aim of encouraging adaptive change is lost because of the negative emotions, such as desire for punishment and revenge, that violence may engender in staff, or because staff may be emotionally drained in the aftermath of an incident. The danger is that if action is taken on the premise that punishment will deter future episodes, it may have the opposite effect through producing anger and resentment in the recipient. In the absence of adequate training and support, staff may interpret the actions of the client as a personal challenge and react 'naïvely', based on emotion rather than considered thought.

■ *Debriefing interview for clients who have become violent*

When   When the available evidence suggests that the aggressor no longer poses an immediate threat and has some degree of self-control. The exact timing requires professional judgement: too soon after an

	incident risks triggering a recurrence; too long may mean that the aggressor's recall is impaired and they may have 'altered' it by 'restructuring' their role in it
Where	A private area that is safe but immediately accessible in case of further aggression
Interviewer	Preferably someone unconnected to the immediate incident who is seen as having a positive relationship with the aggressor and is credible, authoritative and fair.

■ *Process*

The purpose of a debriefing incident is to enable aggressors to gain insight into the causes of their behaviour and to promote the development of alternative adaptive responses. The interview is structured in a series of stages that need to be worked through successively. At each stage, the interviewer attempts to promote the client's understanding of how each stage informs the next.

The interviewer should attempt to gain an insight into the client's perceptions of the situation and the events that transpired before offering alternative perceptions or interpretations, or prompting them from the client. The successive stages of debriefing can be presented alphabetically.

A Antecedents

Exploration of the factors that may have contributed to or triggered the incident. Particular attention should be paid to the client's cognitions and interpretations, and their effect on observable behaviour. Note that antecedents here include 'distal' events – things that may have happened some time before the event – as well as 'proximal' events – things that may have happened immediately before. It also includes as antecedents what the client was thinking and feeling before the incident as well as his or her observable behaviour.

B Behaviour

This covers what the person did, and what he or she felt and thought during the incident as it evolved.

C Consequences

The consequences that resulted from the behaviour:

(a) for the participant
(b) for others.

D Design

The interviewer should attempt to design a plan to aid the aggressor in avoiding a recurrence of the behaviour identified. The plan should include:

(a) The setting conditions for the behaviour (the circumstances in which recurrence might be likely)
(b) The alternative behaviour/cognitions that the aggressor could attempt to employ to prevent recurrence or substitute a more acceptable behaviour
(c) How the person will be helped and by whom
(d) The consequences that will follow recurrence of the aggressive behaviour, and the rewards that will result from the use of alternative acceptable behaviours.

E Enter

Staff members should assist the client in re-engaging in normal activities for that setting.

■ Caveat

Of note with regard to CALM is the clear recognition that some incidents will not involve a linear progression from stage 1 through to stage 6. In practice, it is recognised that some clients may work through the stages in a manner that means they go from stage 1 to stage 2 and then back to stage 1 before moving to 2 and then 3 and so on. It is also recognised that, with some clients who have severe communication difficulties or whose thought processes are severely disordered, a client-based post-incident review may not be practicable. In such a situation, staff should conduct a post-incident review focusing on implications for the future care and management of the client.

■ Post-incident debriefing

Although the research on the effectiveness of post-incident debriefing as a procedure to prevent the development of psychological sequelae (particularly post-traumatic stress disorder) as a consequence of violence or other trauma is ambiguous (Bisson and Deahl 1994), post-incident debriefing for staff assaulted and injured at work can be argued to be a demonstration of care by the organisation for the individual assaulted. It thus, arguably, does not matter whether it is effective in preventing psychological trauma. Post-incident debriefing should routinely follow a incident in which a staff member has been injured or a potentially serious near miss has occurred.

Different perspectives

Both perspectives described share a similar value base. Comparing the two perspectives suggests both marked differences and essential similarities. The focus of the first model is on the immediacy of an incident when aggression is present and violence may be imminent. The CALM model extends de-escalation from the immediacy of a violent incident to encompass both what should happen before an incident and what should happen afterwards as well as what to do during an incident.

In terms of advice for practice in immediate incident management, the primary distinction between CALM and the adapted version of Bailey's model is the attention drawn to the need to consider where the client is on the aggression cycle and how to adjust practice accordingly. The model initially presented, however, advocated a flexible approach based on observation of the client's arousal and response to the actions of staff, which should in turn determine the staff's next actions. The CALM model attempts to ground that 'flexible response' (Turnbull et al. 1990) in theory by providing an explanation of when and why practice should be adjusted, using crisis incident theory as a reference point.

Conclusion

De-escalation cannot and will not prevent all incidents in any given situation of crisis as the actions of a member of staff are only one among a multitude of variables that will affect the outcome in terms of the behaviour of the client. De-escalation can at best still be argued to be an inexact science because each situation is a unique event, and the factors precipitating and maintaining aggression will vary between incidents and during the incident itself. Careful attention to practice can reduce the likelihood of violence, but it will not eliminate it, and even where the practice of staff is exemplary, incidents of violence may still occur. Critical analysis of incidents should be a regular practice, but it must occur within a non-blaming culture in which the aim of the review is to promote learning rather than, either explicitly or implicitly, to apportion blame.

The aim of the preceding review has been to explore what we know about de-escalation and how de-escalation works. Considerable research is still necessary, but significant progress has already been made in moving the practice of de-escalation beyond the realm of intuition.

References

Argyle M (1983) *The Psychology of Interpersonal Behaviour*, London, Penguin.

Averill J.R. (1982) *Anger and Aggression: An Essay on Emotion*, New York, Springer Verlag.

Bailey R.H. (1977) *Violence and Aggression*, The Netherlands (B.V.) Time-Life.

Barlow, D.J. (1989) Therapeutic holding: effective interventions with the aggressive child, *Journal of Psychosocial Nursing*, **27**: 10–14.

Berkowitz L. (1993) *Aggression – Its Consequences, Causes and Control*, McGraw-Hill, New York.

Bisson J.I. and Deahl M. (1994) Psychological debriefing and the prevention of post traumatic stress disorder, *British Journal of Psychiatry*, **165**: 717–20.

Blair D.T. (1991) Assaultive behaviour. Does provocation begin in the front office?, *Journal of Psychosocial and Mental Health Services*, **29**(5): 21–6.

Breakwell G. (1989) *Facing Physical Violence*, Leicester, British Psychological Society.

Breakwell G. and Rowett C. (1989) Violence in social work. In Browne K. (ed.) *Human Aggression Naturalistic Approaches*, London, Routledge.

Burrow S. (1994) Nurse-aid managment of psychiatric emergencies: 3, *British Journal of Nursing*, **3**(3): 121–5.

Conlon L., Gage A. and Hillis T. (1995) Managerial and nursing perspectives on the response to inpatient violence. In Crichton J. (ed.) *Psychiatric Patient Violence: Risk and Response*, London, Duckworth.

Cox T. and Cox S. (1993) *Psychosocial and Organisational Hazards: Control and Monitoring*. Occupational Health Series, No. 5, Copenhagen, World Health Organisation (Europe).

Davies W. (1989) The prevention of assault on professional helpers. In Howell K. and Hollis C.R. (eds) *Clinical Approaches to Violence*, Chichester, John Wiley & Sons.

Farrell G.A. and Gray C. (1992) *Agresion: A Nurse's Guide to Therapeutic Management*, London, Scutari Press.

Fein A.F., Garreri E. and Hansen P. (1981) Teaching staff to cope with patient violence, *Journal of Continuing Education in Nursing*, **12**(2): 21–6.

Gertz B. (1980) Training for prevention of assaultative behaviour in a psychiatric setting, *Hospital and Community Psychiatry*, **31**: 628–30.

Greaves A. (1994) Organisational approaches to the prevention and management of violence. In Whykes T. (ed.) *Violence and Health Care Professionals*, London, Chapman & Hall.

Infantino J. and Musingo S.Y. (1985) Assaults and injuries among staff with and without training in aggression control techniques, *Journal of Hospital and Community Psychiatry*, **32**: 497–8.

Kaplan S.G. and Wheeler E.G. (1983) Survival skills for working with potentially violent clients, *Social Casework*, **64**: 339–45.

La Vigna G. and Donnellan A.M. (1986) *Alternatives to Punishment*, Washington, Irvington.

Leadbetter D. (1993) *Systematic De-escalation of Aggression: An Approach to Risk Management and Behavioural Change for Health and Social Welfare Staff*, Edinburgh, Lothian Regional Council Social Work Department In-Service Training Programme Support Brochure.

Leadbetter D. and Paterson B. (1995) De-escalating aggressive behaviour in management of aggression and violence. In Stark C. and Kidd B. (eds) *Health Care*, London, Gaskell/Royal College of Psychiatrists,.

Leadbetter D. and Trewartha R. (1996) *Handling Aggression and Violence at Work*, Lyme Regis, Russell House Publishing.

Lowe T. (1992) Characteristics of effective nursing interventions in the management of challenging behaviour, *Journal of Advanced Nursing*, **17**(11): 226–32.

MacDonnnell A.A., McEvoy J. and Dearden R.L. (1994) Coping with violent situations in the caring environment. In Whykes T. (ed.) *Violence and Health Care Professionals*, London, Chapman & Hall.

Madden D.J. (1977) Voluntary and involuntary treatment of aggressive patients, *American Journal of Psychiatry*, **134**: 553–5.

Mehrabian A. (1969) *Tactics in Social Influence*, New Jersey, Prentice-Hall.

Mehrabian A. (1972) *Non-verbal Communication*, Chicago, Aldine Atherton.

Morrison E.F. (1990) The tradition of toughness, *Image, Journal of Nursing Scholarship*, **22**(1): 33–5.

Morton P. (1986) Managing assault: your patient is losing control and you're a convenient target, *American Journal of Nursing*, **86**: 1114–16.

Mueller C.W. (1983) Environmental stressors and aggressive behaviour. In Green R.G. and Donnerstein E.I. (eds) *Aggression: Theoretical and Empirical Reviews*, New York, Academic Press.

Negley E.N. and Manley J.T. (1990) Environmental interventions in assaultative behaviour, *Journal of Gerontological Nursing*, **16**: 29–32.

Neizo B.A. and Lanza M. (1984) Post violence dialogue: perception change through language restructuring, *Issues in Mental Health Nursing*, **6**: 245–54.

Novaco R. (1975) *Anger Control: The Development and Evaluation of an Experimental Treatment*, Lexington, DC, Health Co.

Novaco R. (1976) The function and regulation of the arousal of anger, *American Journal of Psychiatry*, **133**: 1124–8.

Novaco R. (1977) Stress inoculation: a cognitive therapy for anger and its application to a case of depression, *Journal of Consulting and Clinical Psychology*, **45**: 600–8.

Paterson B. (1994) Violence and nursing: policy, practice and training, *Advanced Hospital Management*, **3**: 22–5.

Paterson B., Turnbull J. and Aitken I. (1992) An evaluation of a training course in the short-term management of aggression, *Nurse Education Today*, **12**: 368–75.

Rice M.E., Harris G.T. Varney G.W. *et al.* (1990) *Violence in Institutions: Understanding, Prevention and Control*, Toronto, Hoefgre and Huber.

Siann G. (1985) *Accounting for Aggression*, London, Allen & Unwin.

Stark C., Paterson B. and Kidd B. (1995) Incidence of assaults on staff in the NHS, *Nursing Times*, 3 May: 20.

Steadman H.J. (1982) A situational approach to the understanding of violence, *International Journal of Law and Psychiatry*, **5**: 171–86.

Stevenson S. (1991) Heading off aggression with verbal de-escalation, *Journal of Psychosocial Nursing*, **29**: 6–10.

Tardiff K. (1989) *Assessment and Management of Violent Patients*, London, American Psychiatric Press.

Toch H. (1969) *Violent Men: An Inquiry into the Psychology of Violence*, Chicago, Aldine.

Turnbull J., Aitken I. , Black L. and Paterson B. (1990) Turn it around, short-term management of violence and aggression, *Journal of Psychosocial Nursing and Mental Health Services*, **26**(6): 6–12.

Weisfeld G. (1994) Aggression and dominance in a social world. In Archer J. (ed.) *Male Violence*, London, Routledge.

7

MANAGING PHYSICAL VIOLENCE

Brodie Paterson and David Leadbetter

Introduction

Violent behaviour has probably, in some form or other, always been a part of nursing. Its 'rediscovery' over the past 20 years can probably be credited to three main factors:

1. A changing ideological and clinical context, which meant that some of the 'traditional' approaches that may have characterised the management of violence in some settings, particularly the excessive and/or inappropriate use of medication and staff for client violence, were rendered unacceptable (Paterson 1994). This was accompanied by a genuine desire by clinicians and educationalists to improve the quality of care in this area
2. Changing beliefs and values within the wider society about violence (Dobash and Dobash 1992)
3. The influence of Health and Safety legislation and the report of the Health Services Advisory Committee (HSAC) of the Health and Safety Executive (1987).

In Britain, employers have a statutory obligation under the Health and Safety at Work Act to identify the nature and extent of the risk and to devise measures that would provide a safe workplace and a safe system of work. In discharging these responsibilities, it was recommended by the Health Services Advisory Committee of the Health and Safety Executive (1987) that employers:

■ Develop effective policies
■ Provide suitable training for staff and managers, including, where appropriate, training in the physical management of aggression

■ Develop support mechanisms for staff subjected to assault or aggressive behaviour.

The issue of responsibility has been reiterated in the *The Management of Health and Safety At Work Approved Code of Practice* (Health and Safety Commission 1992), which requires employers formally to conduct a risk assessment and to plan and implement a safe system of work, including, where necessary, training (McKay 1994, Stark and Paterson 1994).

Progress

Progress within the United Kingdom in implementing these recommendations is slow and inconsistent. A survey of UK hospitals by the National Union of Public Employees (NUPE 1991) found that only 40 per cent of hospitals had a policy on violence, and a more recent Royal College of Nursing survey of community nurses (Royal College of Nursing 1984) found that only 16.9 per cent of employers had a policy on aggression and violence. These findings may not be representative, but the apparent absence of policy guidance in some areas should give serious cause for concern for a number of reasons:

1. Violence is notoriously under-reported (Morrison 1988). In the absence of a policy, it is likely that no mechanism for reporting violence would exist. This may result in continued 'invisibility' of the problem.
2. There is uncertainty and anxiety about what represents acceptable and legitimate practice. In the absence of clear policy guidance and training in some areas on the specific issue of physical restraint, it is invariably identified as a major source of potential stress, staff alienation and poor practice (Turnbull *et al.* 1990, Miller 1991). Staff fear/uncertainty during incidents can contribute to dysfunctional responses to aggression and may precipitate assaults by staff on clients.
3. Failure to follow good practice may increase the vulnerability to litigation for negligence from service users or staff suffering harmful physical or psychological consequences arising from aggression and violence (Ishimoto 1984, Lanza and Milner 1989, Paterson 1994).

4. The use of *ad hoc* restraint methods or techniques learned in other contexts may increase the risk of injury to all parties. In the absence of training staff, attempting to restrain may expose staff and the client to considerable danger (Paterson *et al.* 1992).

5. An over-reliance may be placed on male staff to manage episodes of aggression (Ryan and Postner 1989). This form of practice is professionally unacceptable as it exposes one group of staff, that is, men, to a disproportionate risk and is probably illegal in that it is contrary to sex discrimination legislation.

Training needs will always vary widely depending on the role and situations of the staff involved. Training should always be based on a training needs analysis that identifies and closely matches the provision of training to identified need (Paterson 1993). It must incorporate research findings, be designed around identified competencies and be carefully evaluated and monitored. The constant review and development of techniques on the basis of the evaluation of operational experience is the vital factor. Physical contact skills cannot and should not be taught in isolation but only as part of an integrated curriculum ensuring that staff have a value base and competencies that limit such physical contact to being a last resort in a violent situation.

The content of training for any staff group must be designed to ensure they are adequately equipped with the appropriate values, knowledge and skills base to practise effectively within their clinical area. The role of staff and thus their requirements for training will vary significantly. Where the remit of any staff member involves the clinical treatment of individuals with a problem of aggression and violence, it is absolutely vital that they are adequately prepared to undertake longer-term therapeutic work with the individual concerned to reduce the likelihood of aggression and violence as well as to safely manage the presenting behaviour in the interim (Goldstein and Keller 1987).

In terms of the historical development of restraint training in Britain, it may be important to briefly describe some key events. The first systematic approach to physically managing violence to become widespread in Britain was Control and Restraint (or as it has become almost universally known C&R), a system developed by the Home Office in the early 1980s for use by the uniformed services, initially the prison service and latterly many police forces. Advantages identified arising from its implementation included (Healy, personal communication, 1993):

- A reduction in the numer of injuries (staff and prisoners)
- A fall in staff sick leave
- Increased staff use of verbal interventions (because of increased confidence)
- The erosion of discriminatory attitudes.

The special hospitals in England, which comprise Broadmoor, Rampton and Ashworth, pioneered the adaptation of C&R programmes developed within the prison service to provide training in the physical management of violence (Tarbuck 1992), and a number of programmes were incorporated into basic and post-basic training in various settings in Scotland (Paterson *et al.* 1992).

The system included a form of wrist lock variously known as the 'gooseneck' or the 'ultimate hold', in which pressure can be applied to the wrist while the elbow is held. Although offering a very secure hold, this wrist lock has the potential to be used and misused as a form of control based on pain compliance. A number of programmes validated by the English National Board have incorporated elements of C&R, principally ENB 955 (The Care of the Violent or Potentially Violent Individual) and ENB 960 (The Principles of Psychiatric Nursing in Secure Environments). The Department of Health guidelines *Permissible Forms of Control in Children's Residential Care* (Department of Health 1993) seemed to many to imply official approval of the system by its use of the term 'Control & Restraint' in its discussion of appropriate training.

Some controversy and confusion about the status of C&R has occurred in some settings. The inquiry led by Louis Blom-Cooper (Department of Health and Special Hospitals Service 1992) into complaints about Ashworth Hospital expressed concern about some elements of C&R as it was being used, particularly with regard to the use of pinch releases or nips. This led to a wide-ranging review of C&R training in the special hospitals, with major changes to the programme content and training strategy. In Aycliffe, a secure children's centre in County Durham where staff had been trained in C&R by prison service trainers, an inquiry was instigated into a number of injuries sustained by young people. However, the subsequent Social Services Inspectorate report (1993) on Aycliffe, *A Place Apart*, confirmed that a number of the injuries had occurred prior to the introduction of C&R and established no links between the injuries sustained by the residents and the methods of restraint taught to the staff. The authors, however, are aware of a number of instances in which the importation of 'unmodified' C&R techniques into health and social care settings has been extremely problematic.

Regrettably, one apparent legacy of the lack of regulation is the confusion that has been allowed to develop around the exact inventory of techniques within specific systems. Given the number of agencies offering restraint training described as C&R or incorporating elements, in various modified forms, of C&R, it is difficult at this point to regard the term 'C&R' as a unitary entity in a national context. Some organisations have developed manuals and protocols and academically and/or professionally accredited instructor training along with internal procedures to review programme content (Forth Valley College 1995). This situation is far from universal, and C&R has arguably, in some respects, become a victim of its own success. The rapidity of its dissemination meant that there were inadequate mechanisms to prevent the development of a plethora of instructor programmes, and an inherently flawed pyramidal training system was thus allowed to develop by default.

There are at least three primary variants and numerous other variants of C&R, between which there are significant differences. The three main variants are:

■ The approach used within the prison services, which themselves vary to some extent between England, Scotland and Northern Ireland
■ The physical control skills element, which forms one part of the 'Care and Control' programmes offered by the English special hospitals who themselves no longer use the term C&R
■ C&R General Services, an adapted version of C&R specifically developed for use in health and social services contexts developed by the originators of C&R, Aiden Healy and Keith Mann.

C&R, in its various manifestations, is probably the most commonly used system in the United Kingdom in health care settings but a variety of other systems are available or may become available shortly. These include:

■ The 'Moran' approach imported from the United States and reportedly used with some success in Argyle and Bute Health board in Scotland (Moran 1984)
■ Therapeutic Crisis Intervention (Badlong et al. 1992), a system developed by Cornell University in the United States and marketed by a number of organisations in the United Kingdom, including the University of Dundee, primarily for child care

- CALM (Crisis Aggression Limitation and Management) developed initially for use in Lothian Region social work department and now used by a number of organisations, including the Scottish Autistic Society and a number of local authorities throughout the United Kingdom
- Strategies for Crisis Intervention and Prevention (SCIP), an American system used widely in New York State and latterly in the United Kingdom by a number of organisations, including Loddon school in Hampshire and a number of NHS Trusts
- Protecting Rights in a Caring Environment (PRICE), a system developed by the prison service for use with children and adolescents.

A brief overview of the components of the various systems and their relative advantages and disadvantages is given in Table 7.1, and contact names and addresses are given at the end of the chapter. Although there is a growing body of systematically obtained evidence on the advantages and disadvantages of various systems (Chadwick 1994, Cran 1995), the qualitative comments reflect the views of the authors in the absence of systematic comparative evaluation. The systems vary widely in content and duration, and information on content for some of them is restricted for security and/or commercial reasons.

There appear to be four essential approaches, which, either singly or in combination, can be used as the basis of any restraint system (Leadbetter 1995). These are:

- The immobilisation of the subject by the use of weight or strength
- The restriction of movement of the long bones by some form of hold or lock
- Maintaining the subject in an off-balance position
- The use of 'reasonable force', which may include pain to encourage compliance.

In the absence of systematic large-scale trials evaluating these competing approaches with respect to the staff's acquisition and retention of skills, safety (in training and practice) for staff and clients, and cost, seven questions are posed that can be asked when attempting to determine the suitability of any approach:

1. Are the techniques being taught effective?
2. Do they contain specific foreseeable risks?

Table 7.1 Description of some systems presently available in the UK

System	Client group	Blocks	Breakaway	Restraint	Relocation
C&R (Control and Restraint Prison)	Adult offenders	Extensive	Extensive	Extensive	Extensive
C&R GS (Control and Restraint General Services)	General health and social care	Extensive	Extensive	Extensive Depends on programme duration	Extensive Depends on programme duration
PRICE (Protecting Rights In a Caring Environment)	Residential child care	Some included	Extensive	Extensive	Included
CALM (Crisis Aggression Limitation and Management)	Children, adolescents, elderly	Extensive	Extensive	Extensive	Extensive
SCIP (Strategies for Crisis Intervention and Prevention)	General health and social care	Extensive	Depends on course length	Depends on course length	Extensive
Care and Responsibility (Ashworth Hospital)	All care settings and industrial adaptations	Extensive Module 1	Extensive Module 1	Extensive Module 2	Extensive Module 2
TCI (Therapeutic Crisis Intervention)	Residential child care	No	Limited	Extensive	Extensive
Moran method	Generic health and social care	No	Limited	Extensive	Extensive

Ethics	Use of pain manual	Accreditation	Updating	De-escalation	Effectiveness
Pain is integral element of the system	Restricted access (Security)	Internal (Home Office)	Formalised arrangement Highly regulated	Integral element of programme	Very effective (requires three-person team for some procedures)
System promotes hierarchical response Pain only as last resort	Full manual to instructors only	Varied depending on delivering agency University of Stirling available	Formalised arrangement Highly regulated	Integral element of programme	Very effective (requires three-person team for some procedures but one and two-person variations)
Described as pain free	None available	None as yet	No formalised arrangement	Integral element of programme	Very effective Phased response
Suggested to be minimal pain	Full manual to instructors only	Centre for Crisis Management	Formalised arrangement Highly regulated	Integral element of programme	Effective range of techniques for one, two, three and four persons
Uses no joints Pain-free	Full manual for Instructors	ENB Portsmouth University Loddon School Bexley Hospital	Formalised arrangement	All programmes include preventative work	Very effective techniques for one to five persons
System designed to minimise use of pain Holding without pain	Full manual to instructors only Handbook for students	Royal College of Nursing and Sheffield Hallam University	Formalised arrangement Highly regulated	Integral element of programme	Very effective (requires three-person team for some procedures but two-person variations)
Suggested to be pain-free	Full manual	Cornell University	No formalised arrangements	Integral element of programme	Effective with younger children
Suggested to be minimal pain	In development	None known in UK	No arrangements	Usually taught as integral element	Effective (not dependent on three-person team)

3. Are the techniques ethical?
4. Are they appropriate for a specific setting?
5. To what degree will the techniques work effectively in situations where staff do not have a strength, height and/or weight advantage?
6. Will the techniques allow me to move someone?
7. Are the techniques legitimate?

Are the techniques taught effective?

As has been suggested, restraint seeks to restore control quickly to an uncontrolled high-risk situation. Therefore, any approach must offer a realistic chance of success, that is, it must actually work in the real world with a highly resistant and aggressive client as well as in controlled simulations. While techniques that claim to be non-invasive are obviously attractive, they will, if they do not actually succeed, inevitably escalate, prolong and complicate a confrontational situation. Immediate compliance by an aggressive and violent person cannot be assumed. Judgements about acceptability and effectiveness must operate from a perspective that incorporates a consideration of a 'worst-case scenario' with the question of resistance in mind.

A confrontation very often involves a process of escalating behaviour. Consequently, it is beneficial if restraint systems offer a selection and hierarchy of responses in which the degree of force or pressure used can be matched to the client's behaviour. This requirement is further underlined by the legal principles that require that any force used be 'reasonable' and the minimum necessary. The use of maximum force involving pain as a first resort is likely to be experienced as abusive. The aim of restraint must be to promote a dialogue, and the maintenance of communication and the ability to easily and progressively relax techniques in line with returning rationality and self-control are, therefore, imperative.

Technically, a number of factors will influence the question of effectiveness. Effective techniques will minimise the client's freedom of movement. The more limbs that are unrestrained, the greater the risk of injury to all parties.

The holds used must be secure. This invariably requires two points of contact with the grasped limb, with the grip closed and the hands opposed.

A crucial judgement involves the question of whether to take the subject to the floor or to restrain in a standing or sitting position. It is probable that, with a strong or very resistant person, floor restraints offer a greater degree of security. 'Flooring', as it is often called, may, however, be experienced by a person as more abusive. MacDonnell *et al.*'s (1993) research on the social acceptability of various restraint methods suggests that observers considered restraint on a chair to be more acceptable than alternatives where the person was held on the floor. It is an absolute essential that if a restraint involves a descent to the floor, the staff member is able to control his/her own balance as there are anecdotal accounts of uncontrolled descents as significant sources of potential injury.

Do they contain specific foreseeable risks?

As George Bernard Shaw suggested, 'The first golden rule may be that there are no golden rules.' No system can offer an unequivocal guarantee of safety where physical contact is involved; there are too many potentially uncontrolled variables and an inadequate research base upon which to draw.

Speculation based on anecdotal evidence suggests commonly reported sources of injury that may be deserving of particular investigation and action to rectify them, including:

- The involvement of inadequate or excessive staff numbers
- The failure to co-ordinate the intervention of staff
- The failure to give explicit protection to the head of the restrained person, particularly in situations where the restrained person is being taken to the ground
- The application of weight or pressure to the chest, back, abdomen or neck
- Failure to control descents.

It is also vital that the safety of the restrained person is not purchased at the expense of that of the staff member. The safety of both staff member and restrained merit equal consideration, and any system must seek to minimise such risks. Members of staff will quickly identify and avoid the use of techniques that are ineffective or result in pain or injury, and that may discredit the physical skills element of any training programme. For example, concerns may be expressed about techniques that ask staff to drop directly on to their knees without being able to use their hands for balance.

Any technique that requires the staff member to be in close proximity to the client's unrestrained limbs certainly presents a foreseeable risk. In general, the greater the restrained person's freedom of movement and the more limbs that are left free, the greater the risk of injury. Training should always include a comprehensive selection of blocking techniques and breakaway techniques that will allow staff to protect themselves and/or escape from situations where necessary.

As with any skill, there is clear evidence that staff competence will diminish over time (Ruane *et al.* 1994). The inoculation view of training, which assumes that attendance on a violence management training course inevitably confers instant and permanent competence, has been discredited, and periodic updating is necessary.

Not all instances of aggression and violence will rapidly resolve themselves. Consequently, in extremis, restraint may need to be sustained over extended periods in order to protect the client or others. It is important, therefore, that the techniques used can minimise physical exertion on the part of the individual being restrained and can avoid placing the client in any position that may cause positional asphyxia. Particularly of concern may be extended periods where clients are held face down, which should be used only with caution where the client is obese or has respiratory problems, where there may be very serious health risks, including sudden death.

The sudden death of a client where the death is associated with violent struggle and restraint may give rise to significant controversy and allegations of abuse (Sheppard 1994). Excluding deaths from natural causes, principally fatal cardiac arrhythmia arising from a combination of pre-existing heart disease and extreme physical exertion, three key factors appear to be associated with such deaths:

- Agitated delirium/acute excited states
- Positional asphyxia
- Neuroleptic therapy.

Acute excited states, or 'agitated delirium' (Bell *et al.* 1992), comprise a phenomenon in which a combination of agitation, aggression and hyperpyrexia occur simultaneously and has been suggested to be associated with sudden death (Mirchandani *et al.* 1994). Such states have been described in cocaine intoxication, but deaths have been reported only where an acute excited delirium psychosis develops; the notion of agitated delirium as a potential cause of death outside such particular circumstances, which are rare in care or custody, has been criticised as unsubstantiated speculation with no theoretical base (New York State Commission of Corrections 1995).

Anxiety has, however, long been associated empirically with an increased risk of fatal myocardial infarction and sudden death (Piccirillo *et al.* 1997). Agitation occurring as a consequence of mental disorder may result in situations in which prolonged exercise may lead to physiological exhaustion without the client experiencing subjective fatigue. The resulting high levels of adrenaline, lactic acidosis and dehydration may increase the susceptibility to cardiac arrhythmia, particularly where a pre-existing medical condition produces a predisposition (Farnham and Kennedy 1997).

Post-mortem examination for death occurring during struggle or restraint must, however, carefully exclude what may be the more likely probability of 'positional asphyxia' (New York State Commission of Corrections 1995), when, as a consequence of the application of restraint, respiration is compromised, causing hypoxia and disturbed heart rhythm (Reay *et al.* 1992). It has been associated with a number of deaths during physical restraint, both with 'mechanical' restraint, in which some garment of equipment is used to restrain an individual (Miles and Irvine 1992, National Law Enforcement Technology Centre 1995), and when no equipment has been used but staff have employed some means of hands-on-technique to physically restrict an individual's freedom of movement.

The available evidence suggests that a combination of factors may place individuals at risk of positional asphyxia. These include position during restraint (particularly face-down prone but also hyperflexion), obesity, a prolonged struggle, drug and alcohol intoxication, mania, respiratory syndromes, including asthma and bronchitis, and cardiovascular disorders (O'Halloran and Lewman 1993).

Of particular concern are restraint positions that may physically mirror a highly dangerous law enforcement practice in some American states of 'hog tying' (see Figure 7.1), most often associated with case reports of positional asphyxia in the literature (Bell *et al.* 1992, National Law Enforcement Technology Centre 1995, Stratton *et al.* 1995). The experimental application of this procedure to non-struggling healthy volunteers dramatically altered their cardio-

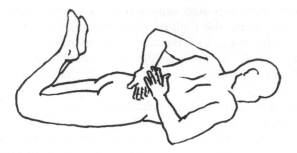

Figure 7.1   Face-down restraint in 'hog-tied' prone position, arms
in hammer lock position with hands resting on back

pulmonary function within 3 minutes (Roeggla *et al.* 1997). Face-
down restraint in the prone position should represent the maximal
permissible intervention in terms of restraint. Its use should be
discouraged where possible and practicable, and restraint in a
seated position or a face-up prone position encouraged. Where face-
down prone restraint is used, attention must be paid to preventing
the possibility of positional asphyxia, particularly for significantly
obese clients, and the subject being restrained should be moved to a
safer position as rapidly as possible.

The role of neuroleptics with respect to sudden death involving
restraint has also been the subject of speculation for some time
(Laposata *et al.* 1988). A number of case reports link neuroleptic
therapy, particularly the phenothiazines, to deaths involving violent
struggle, and Kumar (1997) reviews the potential mechanisms of
death identified, including cardiac arrhythmia and respiratory
failure. The adverse effects of neuroleptic therapy, therefore, represent another variable that may influence or account for sudden
death during restraint.

Where restraint is inevitable, staff involved in restraint procedures must be instructed in the contributory factors that may
influence positional asphyxia. If restraint is a foreseeable event,
risk assessment protocols should routinely identify any
contraindications for particular techniques with particular clients
and ensure that these are communicated to all members of the
clinical team. In addition, staff must be trained to recognise the
early signs of asphyxia and the need for prompt action and urgent
medical attention. Seclusion under constant monitoring, while
unfashionable, may represent a safer alternative to prolonged
restraint for some clients, although this hypothesis is unproved

and sudden deaths have been reported in seclusion subsequent to restraint (Sheppard 1994).

Are the techniques ethical?

This is perhaps the most difficult judgement and an area in which age, gender and cultural factors and the prevalence of past experiences of physical and/or sexual abuse are of fundamental importance and may influence decisions. Where violence is probable, the use of specific methods of restraint should preferably be part of a care plan, although attempts to 'prescribe' methods by providing a detailed description of the exact techniques to be used with individuals is often complicated by the variety of environments in which restraint may need to be initiated.

Some techniques may carry an increased probability of compromising the dignity of participants or mirroring and reinforcing previously distressing experiences involving physical or sexual abuse. From this perspective, a number of techniques may merit particular attention. These include:

- All techniques that involve 'flooring'
- Techniques that involve holding the trunk, for example bear hugs
- Techniques that involve 'straddling' the client on the ground
- Techniques that push a client's face into the floor
- Techniques that may involve pain compliance, such as wrist locks.

Consideration of the issue of pain is central to a discussion on the ethical implications of practice in this area. Some techniques in systems such as the version of C&R used by the prison service use pain (or the potential of self-inflicted pain if the person struggles against the lock or hold) to gain compliance from the individual being restrained. Modified C&R systems emphasise a hierarchical response in which any technique involving pain would only be used as a last resort when an individual could not be controlled by non-painful methods and there was an immediate and serious danger to themselves or others. The use of pain is then justified legally by reference to the concept of reasonable force, and ethically by reference to utilitarianism.

The reality is that some discomfort seems to be almost inevitable in the implementation of restraint. It may range from mild discomfort to severe pain, and it may be an integral element of a programme, a last resort strategy used in the context of reasonable force or an implicit consequence of a particular technique. If we accept the premise that some element of discomfort is involved in all systems and that no system that is without a degree of discomfort actually works, then, in terms of ethical acceptability, the problem is to find a system that is as free of any form of discomfort as possible while retaining maximum effectiveness. This is the 'holy grail' of physical control training, but significant progress has arguably been made in some areas.

There is an ongoing debate on whether it is feasible to restrain effectively without recourse to the use of pain compliance, particularly when the individual being restrained enjoys an advantage in height, weight and/or strength over those who are attempting to restrain him or her. Such situations test the ability of all systems but may particularly pose problems for those who eschew any use of pain in any situation.

Are they appropriate for a specific setting?

A number of issues must be considered here. Nursing is a diverse profession practised across a hugely varying range of settings. It may, therefore, be important to avoid global prescriptions and ensure that specific approaches offer an adequate and realistic response to specific behaviour. Asking staff to employ ineffective or, conversely, over-forceful methods will be unhelpful. The techniques that might be appropriate to deal with a confused and violent woman of 80 years of age suffering from osteoporosis may be different from those necessary to manage the violence of a fit young man with a personality disorder.

Similarly, if training is based on techniques that require a greater number of staff than are actually on duty, the potential for misfortune is obvious. It is no use, for example, training people to operate in a three-person team if there are only two staff on duty at any one time and no reliable means of summoning immediate assistance.

The question of the physical layout of buildings is crucial. For example, incidents may occur in confined spaces such as corridors, or in rooms where there are hard or abrasive floors or solid furnishings such as chairs and tables. In such circumstances, it may be more practical and safe to use techniques that involve standing or sitting restraints rather than those which take the subject to the ground; these, while perhaps offering increased security, may involve a heightened risk of injury.

To what degree will the techniques work effectively in situations where staff do not have a strength, height and/or weight advantage?

In nursing, women form the majority of the staff group, and they may be disproportionately more likely to be assaulted by male clients than their male colleagues (Stark *et al.* 1995). Non-discriminatory practice requires us to ensure that approaches can be mastered by the average employee, and approaches must therefore be based on technique rather than being overly dependent on physical size or strength. It would be both naïve and disingenuous to deny that, over time, a physically stronger individual is likely to prevail over a weaker one, but technique should be the key factor that enables disadvantages in terms of height, weight and strength to be compensated for as far as is possible.

Will the techniques allow me to move someone?

The reality of nursing practice may mean that staff may require as a last resort to move someone against their will safely in a variety of settings for example, in or out of a vehicle, up and down stairs, or through doors. Systems must therefore offer staff the means to do this effectively and safely while maintaining the clients dignity.

Are the techniques legitimate?

Legitimacy with regard to any use of force is a complex issue. Currently, no method carries an unambiguous official endorsement across all contexts. The nearest is Control and Restraint and some of the various adapted versions available. No system can offer a guarantee of legitimacy in that, whenever and wherever force is used, the legitimacy of any given approach or technique will be determined by whether the use of force involved complied with the relevant law specific to the context in which it was used.

Essentially, it appears that two principal criteria must be met (Gostin 1986):

1. There must be a legitimate reason to use force.
2. The force used must be demonstrably 'reasonable'.

In considering legitimacy, a variety of reasons considered legitimate to justify the use of force occur in law. (It should be noted that there are major variations in law between some member countries of the United Kingdom, and this subject is explored in more depth in Chapter 4).

Five main categories may be suggested to apply (Hoggett 1985, 1990), all of which are only legitimate on the premise that no other option is available:

- The prevention of a crime
- The prevention of a breach of the peace
- Self-defence (The law imposes a duty on a potential victim to retreat and escape, and it is only where no opportunity to disengage is available that self-defence is likely to be considered legitimate [Martin 1990])
- The restraint of a 'dangerous lunatic' (There is no suggestion that this is an appropriate term to use, and a modern interpretation of this concept would generally include those individuals covered under the term 'mental disorder' used in both the Mental Health Act 1983 and the Mental Health (Scotland) Act 1984)
- In certain contexts, the authority to use force may be derived from specific legislation, such as the Mental Health Act 1983 or Mental Health (Scotland) Act 1984.

Reasonable force

Even where the law provides a potentially legitimate reason for the use of force, any force used must be able to meet the criteria of 'reasonableness' (Gostin 1986). The concept of reasonableness is complex and can only in any given instance be absolutely determined by a court of law (Lyon 1994). Reasonableness in this context has, however, been defined thus: 'the force used should be no more than was necessary to accomplish the object for which it is allowed (so retaliation, revenge and punishment are not permitted) and second, the reaction must be in proportion to the harm which is threatened' (Dimond 1990).

An example of an illegitimate and unreasonable use of force would be to strike someone in retaliation after an assault. An example of a potentially legitimate and reasonable use of force would be physically to hold an individual who was detained under Mental Health Act legislation and noted to be suicidal to prevent an ongoing attempt by the person to throw him or herself under the wheels of moving car until that car, and thus the immediate danger, had passed. Unfortunately, between these relatively clear-cut examples, there are a number of grey areas. Is it legitimate to use force, for example, to prevent a confused elderly man leaving a nursing home to go for a walk because you consider that he is at risk of being knocked down in a road traffic accident? Is it legitimate to intervene using force to restrain a client who is destroying furniture but not threatening his or her own safety or that of members of staff or other clients?

The use of risk assessment where the potential of harm arising from an event is established can provide a tool to identify a reasonable response and should be used routinely where evidence indicates the potential or actual use of restraint.

Self-defence training

The issue of training in self-defence as opposed to the systems previously described is potentially fraught with even more difficulty. MacDonnell et al. (1994) have described 'a frightening degree of variability in training and teacher competence'. There is little consistency between approaches and within certain systems there are techniques that are explicitly designed to inflict the maximum possible damage on an attacker. The inherent philosophy of many self-defence programmes seems at odds with that required within health and social care contexts, where the concern is to attempt to protect both the victim and the potential assailant from injury. Accordingly, the possibility of their importation must be viewed with real concern with regard to the potential consequences. Techniques from self-defence training intended specifically to seriously harm an assailant, such as gouging the eyes with the fingers, may play a part in extreme emergencies where attempts to block and/or break away from attack have failed and mortal danger is present, but there must be grave concerns when these approaches are not placed within the context of a hierarchical response that advocates techniques designed to cause minimum harm first.

Does training work?

There are regrettably few published studies describing or evaluating programmes intending to equip nurses with the necessary skills to practise in this area. In general, staff participating in such courses evaluated them positively (Fein *et al.* 1981), and there is some evidence that certain programmes contributed to reductions in the number of recorded incidents and in levels of stress and burnout among staff (Infantino and Musingo 1985, Rice *et al.* 1989, Goodykoontz and Herrick 1990). There have also been suggestions that training in aggression and violence management may generally be associated with a decrease in the risk of assault and injury (Rosenthal *et al.* 1992).

However, an extremely wide variation in programme content and duration (Robinson and Barnes 1986), together with an inadequate description of programme content in the studies (Wong 1992) and alleged methodological weaknesses in some studies (Green 1990), makes it difficult to establish definitive conclusions on the effectiveness of such training (Paterson *et al.* 1992). There are even suggestions that some training programmes may be inadequate or even dangerous, carrying an excess risk of injury to participants during training (Tarbuck 1992, Leadbetter 1994).

Conclusion

It would not be appropriate to end this review of the literature on a note of pessimism, even if, with hindsight, we may regret the unregulated market that has been allowed to develop in this area. The literature suggests that, where the realities and demands of coping with challenging behaviour have been recognised and owned at all levels within an agency, many organisations have been able to develop policies and implement training strategies in violence management and physical restraint that have reduced injury and sickness levels and improved practice. Utilising existing staff expertise and involving service users in the discussion are important. The development of appropriate methods of restraint that can be customised to most contexts is technically feasible; the problem is one of will and resources rather than of techniques.

There have been a number of initiatives in this area that are worthy of note. The RCN Institute of Advanced Nursing Education has developed an outline curriculum for instructors in C&R, and

142

some C&R instructors in England and Wales have attempted to collaborate to establish standards for curriculum content and instructor accreditation. The Multi Sectoral Special Interest Group in Violence and Aggression Management Training established in Scotland (MIGVAMT) has published guidelines for purchasers of training. In a recent venture, the Centre for Crisis Management, a registered charity with which the two authors of this chapter have some involvement, has been established to promote collaboration between experts in the establishment of criteria for the accreditation of both systems and instructors. There is also a small but growing body of systematically obtained evidence on the advantages and disadvantages of various systems (Chadwick 1994).

The primary issues outstanding remain the conduction of adequate evaluations of available systems/methods of restraint, including a comparative analysis of different systems and their relative effectiveness in different contexts. A parallel can be drawn between safe practice in restraint and driving. You can approach both in two ways. You can either increase safety by good tuition and constant practice, or you can also produce safer cars by learning from controlled experiment accidents via biomechanical evaluation, and real-life accidents via incident investigation, which will allow identified dangers to be minimised. Experience and logic dictate that both approaches are necessary. Good design based upon good research, including a biomechanical evalaution of the potential risks of techniques, is the vital starting point upon which to base the selection of appropriate techniques used in training. Ongoing development means learning from the system in implementation. In order to so, the implementation of systems must be rigorously monitored, accidents and injuries being reported and scrutinised for their implications for training and practice.

If we are to reduce unsafe *ad hoc* practices, we must ensure that they are replaced by approaches that managers, staff and service users regard as better and safer. There are few instant or easy solutions to the problem of ensuring acceptable practice. While managers and trainers may still be held accountable in the event of an injury, a responsible and systematic approach to the evaluation and regulation of the individual techniques approved for use will be the most potent and effective response to concerns.

References

Badlong M., Holden M. and Mooney A. (1992) *National Residential Childcare Project – Therapeutic Crisis Intervention*, Cornell University, Family Life Development Centre, College of Human Ecology.

Bell M.D., Rao V.J. and Wetli C.V. (1992) Positional asphyxia in adults: a series of 30 cases from the Dade and Broward County, Florida, Medical Examiners Office from 1992–1990, *American Journal of Forensic Medical Pathology*, **13**: 101–7.

Chadwick J. (1994) *Restraint Monitoring Children and Families Services*, Devon Social Services.

Cran J. (1995) *Social Work Services Risk Assessment*, Central Regional Council, Stirling.

Department of Health (1993) *Permissible Forms of Restrasint in Children's Residential Care*, London, DoH.

Department of Health and Special Hospitals Authority (1992) *Report of the Committee of Inquiry into Complaints about Ashworth Hospital* (Blom-Cooper Report) London, HMSO.

Dimond B. (1990) *Legal Aspects of Nursing*, London, Prentice-Hall.

Dobash E.R. and Dobash R. (1992) *Women, Violence and Social Change*, London, Routledge.

Farnham F.R. and Kennedy H.G. (1997) Acute excited states and sudden death, *British Medical Journal*, **315**: 1007–108.

Fein A.F., Garreri E. and Hansen P. (1981) Teaching staff to cope with client violence, *Journal of Continuing Education in Nursing*, **12**(2): 21–6.

Forth Valley College (1995) Instructor manual, *Therapeutic Management of Aggression and Violence/Control and Restraint General Services*, Falkirk, Forth Valley College.

Goldstein A.P. and Keller H. (1987) *Aggressive Behaviour: Assessment and Intervention*, Oxford, Pergamon.

Goodykoontz L. and Herrick C.A. (1990) Evaluation of an in service training programme regarding aggressive behaviour in a psychiatric unit, *Journal of Continuing Education in Nursing*, **21**(3): 77–83.

Gostin L. (1986) *Institutions Observed: Towards a New Concept of Secure Provision in Mental Health*, London, King Edward's Hospital Fund for London.

Green R. (1990) Reducing staff injuries, *Hospital and Community Psychiatry*, **41**(10): 1141–2.

Health and Safety Commission (1992) *The Management of Health and Safety at Work Approved Code of Practice*, London, HMSO.

Health Service Advisory Commission of the Health and Safety Executive (1987) *Violence to Staff in the Health Service*, London, HMSO.

Hoggett B. (1985) Legal aspects of secure provision. In Gostin L. (ed.) *Secure Provision*, London, Tavistock.

Hoggett B. (1990) *Mental Health Law*, 3rd edn, London, Sweet & Maxwell.

Infantino J. and Musingo S.Y. (1985) Assaults and injuries among staff with and without training in aggression control techniques, *Journal of Hospital and Community Psychiatry*, **32**: 497–8.

Ishimoto W. (1984) Security management for health care administrators, in Turner J.T. (ed.) *Violence in the Medical Care Setting: A Survival Guide*, Aspen, CO, Aspen.

Kumar A. (1997) Sudden unexplained death in a psychiatric client – a case report: the role of the phenothiazines and physical restraint, *Medicine, Science and The Law*, **37**(2): 170–5.

Lanza M.L. and Milner J. (1989) The dollar cost of client assault, *Hospital and Community Psychiatry*, **34**: 44–7.

Laposata E.A., Hale P. Jr and Polkis A. (1988) Evaluation of sudden death in psychiatric clients with special reference to phenothiazine therapy: forensic pathology, *Journal of Forensic Science*, **33**: 432–40.

Leadbetter D. (1994) Need for care over methods of restraint, *Community Care*, 18–24 August: 13.

Leadbetter D. (1995) Technical aspects of physical restraint. In Lindsay M. (ed.) *Physical Restraint Practice, Legal, Medical and Technical Considerations*, Glasgow, Centre For Residential Child Care, University of Strathclyde.

Lyon C. (1994) *Legal Issues Arising from the Care Control and Safety of Children with Learning Disabilities who also Present with Challenging Behaviour*, London, Mental Health Foundation.

MacDonnell A.A., Sturmey P.S. and Dearden R.L. (1993) The acceptability of physical restraint procedures, *Behavioural and Cognitive Psychotherapy*, **21**(3): 255–64.

MacDonnnell A.A., McEvoy J. and Dearden R.L. (1994) Coping with violent situations in the caring environment. In Whykes T. (ed.) *Violence and Health Care Professionals*, London, Chapman & Hall.

McKay C. (1994) Violence to health care professionals: a health and safety perspective. In Whykes T. (ed.) *Violence and Health Care Professionals*, London, Chapman & Hall.

Martin A. (1990) The case for self-defence, *Health and Social Service Journal*, **88**: 697.

Miles S.H. and Irvine P. (1992) Deaths caused by physical restraints, *Gerontologist*, **32**(6): 762–6.

Miller R. (1991) Hitting back, *Nursing Times*, **87**(5): 57–8.

Mirchandani H.G., Rorke L.B., Sekula-Perlman A. and Hood K. (1994) Cocaine-induced agitated delirium, forceful struggle and minor head injury. A further definition of sudden death during restraint, *American Journal of Forensic Medical Pathology*, **15**: 95–9.

Moran, J. (1984) Aggression management: response and responsibility, *Nursing Times*, **80**(14): 28–31.

Morrison E.F. (1988) Instrumentation issues in the measurement of violence in psychiatric inclients, *Issues in Mental Health Nursing*, **9**: 9–16.

National Law Enforcement Technology Centre (1995) *Positional Asphyxia-Sudden Death*, Washington, US Department of Justice.

New York State Commission of Corrections (1995) *Dispelling the Myth: 'Sudden in custody death syndrome'*, Chairman's Memorandum No. 14–95, New York State Commission of Correction.

Norris D. (1990) *Violence Against Social Workers. The Implications for Practice*, London, Jessica Kingsley.

NUPE (1991) *Violence in the NHS*, London, NUPE.

O'Halloran R.L. and Lewman L.V. (1993) Restraint asphyxiation in excited delirium, *American Journal of Forensic Medical Pathology*, **14**: 289–95.

Paterson B. (1993) Guidelines for conducting a training needs analysis. In *The Management of Aggression and Violence*, Paisley, Multi Sectoral Special Interest group in Aggression and Violence Management Training.

Paterson B. (1994) Violence and nursing: policy, practice and training, *Advanced Hospital Management*, **3**: 22–5.

Paterson B., Turnbull J. and Aitken I. (1992) An evaluation of a training course in the short term management of aggression, *Nurse Education Today*, **12**: 368–75.

Paterson B., Stark C. and Leadbetter D. (1994) Guidelines on purchasing training in the management of aggression and violence. In *Aggression and Violence Management Training*, Paisley, Multi Sectoral Special Interest Group.

Piccirillo G., Santagada E., Bucca C. *et al.* (1997) Abnormal passive head-up tilt test in subjects with symptoms of anxiety power spectral analysis study of heart rate and blood pressure, *International Journal of Cardiology*, **60**: 121–31.

Reay D.T., Fligner A.D., Stilwell A.D. and Arnold J. (1992) Asphyxia during law enforcement transport, *American Journal of Forensic Medical Pathology*, **13**: 90–7.

Rice M.E., Harris G.T., Varney G.W. and Quinsay V.L. (1989) *Violence in Institutions: Understanding, Prevention and Control*, Toronto, Hoefgre and Huber.

Robinson S. and Barnes J. (1986) Continuing education in relation to the prevention and management of violence. In Wilson-Barnett J. and Robinson S. (eds) *Directions in Nursing Research*, London, Scutari Press.

Roeggla M., Wagner A., Muellner M. *et al.* (1997) Cardio respiratory consequences to hobble restraint, *Wiener Klinische Wochenschrift*, **109**(10): 359–61.

Rosenthal T.L., Edwards N.B., Rosenthal R.H. and Ackerman B.J. (1992) Hospital violence: site, severity and nurse's preventative training, *Issues In Mental Health Nursing*, **13**(4): 349–56.

Royal College of Nursing (1994) *Violence and Community Nursing Staff: A Royal College of Nursing Survey*, RCN, London.

Ruane M., Eaton Y., McAuliffe J. *et al.* (1994) Care and Responsibility Training Skills: Diminution and Retention Study, Unpublished paper, Ashworth Hospital Mental Health Nursing Forensic Practice Development Centre.

Ryan J.A. and Postner E.C. (1989) The assaulted nurse: short term and long term responses, *Archives of Psychiatric Nursing*, **3**: 323–31.

Sheppard D. (1994) *Learning the Lessons: Mental Health Inquiry Reports Published in England and Wales between 1969–1994 and their Recommendations for Improving Practice*, London, Zito Trust.

Social Services Inspectorate (1993) *A Place Apart*, London, Social Services Inspectorate.

Stark C. and Paterson B. (1994) Violence at work, *British Medical Journal*, **308**: 62–3.

Stark C., Paterson B. and Kidd B. (1995) Incidence of assaults on staff in the NHS, *Nursing Times*, May 3: 20.

Stratton S.J., Rogers C. and Green K. (1995) Sudden death in individuals in hobble restraints during paramedic transport, *Annals of Emergency Medicine*, **25**: 710–12.

Tarbuck P. (1992) Use and abuse of control and restraint, *Nursing Standard*, **6**(52): 30–2.

Turnbull J. (1993) Victim support, *Nursing Times*, **89**(23): 33–4.

Turnbull J., Aitken I., Black L. and Paterson B. (1990) Turn it around, short term management of violence and aggression, *Journal of Psychosocial Nursing and Mental Health Services*, **26**(6): 6–12.

Wong E.W. (1992) Violence prevention and the literature, *Journal of Hospital and Community Psychiatry*, **44**: 1158–200.

Addresses

UK contact addresses for systems described. Some systems are available via a number of organisations. The intending purchaser should always investigate alternative systems and, where possible, providers.

Crisis Aggression Limitation and Management (CALM)
Centre for Crisis Management
12 School Lane, Menstrie
Clackmannanshire FK11 7BB

Control and Restraint (C&R)
Mick Traynor
C&R National Trainer
Prison Services Training Services
C&R National Centre
Bawtry Road
Hatfield Woodhouse
Doncaster DN7 6PQ

Control and Restraint – General Services (C&R GS)
Aiden Healy
Home Farm
High Hutton
Huttons Ambo
York YO6 7HN

Control and Restraint General Services (C&R GS) Scottish/Irish contact
Brodie Paterson
Lecturer
Department of Nursing and Midwifery
University of Stirling
Forth Valley Campus
Westburn Avenue
Falkirk FK1 5ST

Care and Responsibility Programmes
Tom Swan
Ashworth Centre
Ashworth Hospital
Parkbourne
Maghull
Liverpool L31 1HW

Moran System
David Bertin
Senior Nurse Manager
Isla Centre
Argyle and Bute Hospital
Lochgilphead
Argyle PA31 8LQ

Protecting Rights In a Caring Environment (PRICE)
Mick Traynor
C&R National Trainer
Prison Services Training Services
C&R National Centre
Bawtry Road
Hatfield Woodhouse
Doncaster DN7 6PQ

Therapeutic Crisis Intervention (TCI)
Martha Holden
Senior Extension Associate
Family Life Development Center
G-20 Van Rensselaer Hall
Ithaca
New York 14853-4401

Strategies for Crisis Intervention and Prevention (SCIP)
Kevin Bond
Mental Health
Services Manager
Dacorum and St Albans
West Herts Community Health
NHS Trust
Mental Health Services
99 Waverly Road
St Albans
Hertfordshire AL3 5TL

8

PROVIDING STAFF WITH ADEQUATE SUPPORT: HEALTH WORKERS AS SURVIVORS OF ASSAULT AND AGGRESSION

Vaughan Bowie

Introduction

This chapter will explore the impact of violence on health care workers and discuss how best to provide support to staff who may experience violence at work both before and after incidents. The small but growing research and observational evidence available on the response of health service workers to assault and violence shows that their reactions parallel those of assaulted non-health service workers. It is also noteworthy that the reaction of significant others, including their own colleagues, often contains the same negative and unhelpful elements as the reactions of non-service workers to peers who are assaulted (Rowett 1986).

Disaster workers and related human service workers often face 'aggression' from natural or man-made calamities but not generally from the clients or patients they are trying to help. However, health service workers who are involved in more direct daily contact with patients are much more vulnerable to verbal or physical attacks by them. While, with face-to-face helpers, a crisis response may occur as the result of any traumatic stress, the stress caused by verbal and physical assault by patients may have some unique effects. Jannoff-Bulman (1992, p. 80) summarises this impact: 'Victimisations that do not involve perpetrators are apt to be humbling, whereas human-induced victimisations are more appropriately characterised as humiliating'. This 'humiliation' involves the following.

First, it is often sudden, arbitrary, unexpected and unpredictable. Its lack of predictability and apparent randomness often gives assaulted staff members no time to erect psychological and physical defences. They may be forced into a reactive, helpless coping pattern.

Second, an attack may cause staff members to lose a sense of control over their life and physical being, sometimes only for seconds but on occasions for hours. No longer do they feel in control of themselves.

Third, although the attack may indeed have been arbitrary, workers may feel chosen for the attack and blame themselves for attracting the attacker. They find it difficult within their world view to accept their assault as a random event.

Fourth, the professional training and socialisation of health service workers emphasises being competent and in control, and makes it extremely difficult and confusing for them when placed in a dependent, victim role. Mitchell (1984, p. 28) expresses this well:

They were trained only to be helpers, not victims. The necessity to be both helper and victim generally produces a psychological conflict that makes people particularly vulnerable to stress reactions, which are characterised by severe fatigue, confusion, denial and withdrawal.

For health services workers, the crisis of a verbal or physical assault may be accompanied by a number of losses and the destruction of cherished beliefs (see Jannoff-Bulman 1992). These losses can include:

- A loss of control of one's life, present and future
- A loss of trust in God or other people
- A loss of a sense of a just and fair world
- A loss of a self-image of being worthwhile
- A loss of a sense of invulnerability and immortality.

Responses of health services staff to verbal and physical assault

As indicated above, health service workers may have three types of shared assumption about themselves and the world shattered by verbal and physical assault:

- The belief in their own invulnerability
- Their perception of the world as a meaningful and comprehensible place – a just world
- That they are worthy decent people, because of respect of others, and have high self-esteem.

As with other survivors, health service workers respond to the shattering of these assumptions following assault with a variety of emotional and physical responses (Whykes and Whittington 1994). Anger, fear or depression can emerge, making a return to work, or an ongoing helpful attitude, difficult to maintain.

Because of such feelings, workers may insist on the discharge, referral or breaking of contact with a violent patient or client. If assaulted, staff feel that outward expression of their anger or fear is not allowed or is inappropriate, they may find indirect methods of expressing their feelings or redirecting them elsewhere, perhaps against other patients, family or staff. These feelings may also be directed against the organisation, its management and safety procedures.

Often, if the outward expression of these emotions is blocked, a sense of frustration, powerlessness and depression may increase. Lenehan and Turner (1984) have noted that symptoms of clinical depression are common among health service workers after a violent incident. Symptoms noted have included sadness and crying spells, feelings of worthlessness and emptiness, lack of direction and motivation, fatigue, irritability, and sleep and eating disturbances.

Lanza (1983), in a study of 40 assaulted nurses' reactions to trauma, noted two major patterns. First, the reactions to assault can last much longer than the time they have off as a result of an assault. Some of Lanza's subjects reported many of the same symptoms as Lenehan and Turner, reported above. Second, however, assaulted staff frequently reported no reaction to the trauma or attempted to rationalise their reactions. As previously mentioned, this 'non-reaction' may be due to denial of vulnerability, desensitisation to the dangers of the job and professional socialisation. Another factor may be their assumption that the health service will do nothing even if they report the incident.

It has been suggested by a number of authors that a great amount of under-reporting of assaults against health staff occurs. Some would suggest for every incident recorded, five or more similar events go unreported (Bowie 1996).

A similar study by Ryan and Poster (1989) of 61 assaulted nursing staff had two major findings. First was that 82 per cent of the assaulted staff felt that they had resolved the crisis caused by the assault within 6 weeks of the incident. However, during that 6-week period, they experienced a variety of physical and emotional responses while attempting to maintain therapeutic relationships with assaultive and other patients. Anger was noted as the staff's main short-term emotional response.

Second, some assaulted staff continued to experience moderate-to-severe reactions 6 months and 12 months after the assault. Such reactions did not necessarily reflect a severe physical assault. Some of these respondents displayed chronic or delayed post-traumatic stress disorder as a result of either the assault or other non-related previous traumatic life events.

Studies of the London Ambulance Service (Ravenscroft 1994) indicated that 15 per cent of the front-line staff reported symptoms consistent with acute post-traumatic stress disorder and as many as 52 per cent were suffering from high levels of stress or recent mental disturbance. Interestingly, the officers reported that the stress they experienced did not come from the major disasters that they attended but had its origins more in shift work, lack of communication with management, privatisation and under-funding, lack of meal breaks and the cumulative strain of responding to routine emergency calls.

Effects of assault of workers on significant others

An 'illusion of semi-invulnerability' protects most of us from the stress and anxiety associated with the threat of assault or violence. This illusion, however, is seriously threatened when someone close to us or a member of a work, family or other personal or social group is assaulted.

At a time when social support needs are critical, survivors of assault may find themselves socially isolated, not only because they might be depressed and unhappy individuals, but also because their presence is often an unwanted reminder to others of their own vulnerability.

Social support for assaulted workers might also be minimised because they are seen as losers or the assault may be perceived by others as 'only a minor verbal encounter'. Assumptions regarding a just world (Lerner 1980) are very powerful, and such assumptions imply that assaulted staff are responsible for their fate and thus deserving of blame and derogatory comments rather than empathy and support.

Significant others in the life of the assaulted staff member may fend off insecurities about their own possible vulnerability by blaming the assaulted staff member for what has befallen them. Jannoff-Bullman (1992, p. 150) illustrates this phenomenon:

> Non victims are motivated to blame victims so that they may continue to maintain their core assumptions about the nature of the world and themselves, and a secondary benefit of such blame is the minimisation of any responsibility and any need they have to help.

Interesting research by Lanza (1987) suggests that nurses who suffer only 'mild' assault may be blamed more than those perceived as receiving a more 'severe' assault, and female staff will receive more blame than male staff. Men also appeared to place blame more heavily on the victim than their female counterparts. Furthermore, age also affected the placement of blame with advancing age increasing the trend to blame colleagues who were assaulted.

Blaming the 'staff victim' assists other staff members to distance themselves from the possibility of themselves also being violated. Thus the assaulted staff member may be labelled by others as unprofessional, aggressive, careless or angry. This retraumatisation may be as devastating to the worker as the original trauma.

A further cause of concern is recent research showing that nursing colleagues are not only unsupportive, but also often identified by assaulted nurses as the major source of verbal and sometimes physical attack (Farrell 1997). This phenomenon is referred to as horizontal violence (Duffy 1995).

Even where workers want to be supportive to an assaulted colleague, there are certain problems that must be faced and overcome. Levy and Brown (1984) note five possible major barriers to a helper's ability to deal with an assaulted person. These five barriers may also be present between staff and colleague helper. The five barriers are:

- A lack of objectivity
- A lack of skills
- A lack of understanding
- A lack of confidence
- Environmental barriers.

Helpers experiencing a lack of objectivity may find that their feelings about their colleague interfere with appropriate responses. Helpers lacking skills may not be able to deal with the issues involved or understand their fellow workers' particular needs and feelings. This may, in turn, lead to a lack of confidence in their ability to be supportive to an assaulted worker. Added to these barriers may be environmental barriers such as agency policy, procedures or lack of resources.

Responding to staff support needs

In responding to the issue of violence against health service workers, there are a number of important issues to be examined. Perhaps the most crucial of these is simply whose responsibility it is to deal with the threat or actual acts of violence.

One response to this question is to suggest that all those involved or potentially involved in the situation must accept some responsibility. These include the patient and the patient's family; the assaulted worker, his or her colleagues and family; and the agency and its administration. It is thus appropriate that both interventive and preventive strategies take into account these differing, and potentially conflicting, perspectives.

It is also clear that responding to the issue of violence against health service workers must address the three interlocking issues of violence prevention, diffusion and post-trauma support for assaulted staff. Thus response strategies must include aspects of education and training, as well as forward planning and the capacity for a quick response during crisis situations, together with ongoing support for the staff survivors of violence.

Individual responses

In the light of the above information, how do health service workers overcome the impact of such traumatic events individually, as a team and within the health services?

Jannoff-Bulman (1985, 1992) and Jannoff-Bulman *et al.* (1983) suggest that there are two main types of personal coping strategy used by victims in order to overcome these losses:

- Intrapsychic/cognitive responses
- Direct action or behavioural responses.

Intrapsychic responses

Such responses are the emotional and psychological reactions to trauma and may include the following.

Redefining the event

Rationalisations may be used that involve comparing the self with others who were much worse off as victims, or by trying to perceive some lesson, experience or benefit that might be gained from the event. Additionally, attempts may be made to explain away or re-appraise the severity of the event or to find some type of meaning or purpose behind it. If some sense of purpose can be found, victims can begin to re-establish a belief in an orderly, understandable world.

Self-blame

Another common cognitive mechanism staff use in an attempt to re-appraise an assault on them is self-blame. In blaming themself for their assault, individuals may make a variety of attributions, and attribution theory would make predictions about the emotional and behavioural consequences of specific attributions. For example, blaming one's character as the reason for being attacked might lead to a sense of hopelessness about the future and would initially appear somewhat maladaptive. However, Kahn (1984) suggests that such self-blame can be quite functional, especially if blame is placed on actions rather than personality. Thus the acceptance of behavioural responsibility provides an individual with 'agenda control' (Peterson and Seligman, 1983), that is, a sense of control over the planning, choosing and changing of contingencies in his or her life.

Behavioural blame can be a particularly effective intervention as it addresses the three major assumptions that have been shattered, namely invulnerability, meaning and self-esteem. Victims can once again believe in some control over, and protection from, events. They are also given some reason for the event occurring, and why they behaved that way, and an opportunity once again to build a positive self-image.

However, if the events are seen as unpredictable or beyond the individual's control, such self-blame approaches will be of little use.

Direct action responses

Direct action responses by assaulted staff can further rebuild the shattered assumptions of invulnerability, meaning and self-esteem. Direct action may provide a renewed sense of control over the immediate environment and serve to minimise the victim's new sense of vulnerability as well as helping re-establish a view of the world as being somewhat responsive to an individual's efforts. Such perceptions of control also help to redevelop a positive self-image and a positive sense of one's own abilities and autonomy.

Direct action can include reporting an offence, taking legal action, increasing security, lobbying for organisational change, moving location, taking self-defence classes or further training.

It can also include seeking social support. Establishing or re-establishing support networks further enables traumatised staff to redevelop basic assumptions about their own self-worth, while also seeing parts of the world, at least, as benevolent again. The failure to receive such support or have it given in an unacceptable fashion may again lead to 'secondary trauma'.

Support

Let us define support a little more clearly. 'Support' is a process of helping and encouraging people so that their work can be done more effectively. It is also a means of providing an emotional buffer against the demands and traumas faced on the job. Kahn and Earle (1982, p. 116) describe this in more detail:

> The support which professional staff should receive from their superiors, supervisors, and colleagues will... depend upon the ready availability of additional skills as well as time. In this situation support is not just encouragement and reassurance, nor is it collusive approval of whatever might happen to have been done. Support requires some discriminations to the value of any alternative decisions and, therefore, it requires the ability to make a professional appraisal of the activities being undertaken. Support also includes the caring for the worker as an individual and as a member of a service, and someone with whom it is worth spending time.

We are not talking here of long-term therapeutic intervention for staff who are suffering from some type of chronic post-traumatic stress. Support should be used as an adjunct to therapeutic interventions.

The need for support can arise because of:

- Isolation
- Unclear aims
- Confused feelings and discouragement
- Difficult communication
- Lack of ideas
- Overwork
- Reduced resources
- Verbal and physical assault at work.

A good support system should be able to supply the following resources. However, they rarely can be found in just one or two people or a supervisor, and there may be dangers in trying to combine all these support functions in just a few people. It is often neither possible nor advisable to seek all these support needs in just one or two people or from the one location. 'Supporters' should come from both workplace and broader family and social contexts whenever possible.

A comprehensive support network (Pines *et al.* 1981) provides the following:

1. *Active listening*
2. *Technical appreciation*
   Someone who can offer technical, how-to-do-it advice and confirm the worker's skills. It requires an expert in their field and someone of honesty and integrity.
3. *Technical challenge*
   Someone who challenges current ways of thinking and stimulates greater exertion and creativity; this again requires expertise and trust.
4. *Emotional support*
   Someone who is on a person's side during times of difficulty, even if he or she is not necessarily in total agreement with that person's actions. Such a person cares more about the individual than his or her position, work or current emotional state.
5. *Emotional challenge*
   Someone who offers the other the opportunity to grow emotion-

ally, using logic to help the individual cut through his or her own emotionality in order to arrive at a rational solution.

6. *Shared social realities*

In times of stress, when one needs sound advice that can be trusted, a person with similar priorities, values and views can be very supportive. A person with a shared world view is most likely to give useful advice.

It is crucial that the support function of colleagues be separated in time and purpose from an investigatory, incident review role. When a staff member is feeling most vulnerable after an assault, it is not helpful to subject them to an investigation, sometimes with implied blame for the incident. The support person(s) should be different from those investigating and reporting on the event for the organisation. This does not mean that the basic 'paperwork' has to be neglected, but it must be done sensitively. Some assault incident forms imply blame, with questions such as 'What would you do differently next time?', and such insensitive questions may lead to secondary trauma.

Both immediate practical and emotional support are needed during and immediately after the trauma and may involve a number of sources of support. For some, these support needs may diminish over the next few months; for others, such support may be needed for 6 months or more.

Blocks to receiving support

The amount of support that a worker actually receives depends upon the availability, accessibility and acceptability of the support, that is, how much, how easily is it gained and how acceptable it is. The support available is often very limited, difficult to access when needed and more orientated to the organisation's needs rather than those of the traumatised staff.

Smythe, in *Surviving Nursing* (1984), suggests that there are a number of blocks to gaining such needed support.

Personal blocks

Health professionals often think that needing help from others is a sign of weakness and non-professionalism, so do not ask for it. This approach is maintained through a conspiracy of silence by other staff.

Also, some administrators view nurses who voice real concerns about safety issues as being troublemakers who need to be removed or diverted. Nursing staff may fear that acknowledging concerns may lead to attack by the administration.

An inability to communicate their support needs or the uncertainty of what type of support they need may also be blocks to people gaining support. Fear of rejection because of low self-esteem or negative past responses may also be a reason for not seeking or accepting support.

Professional blocks

Some of the professional blocks to gaining support centre on issues such as the level and type of professional training received, the use of temporary staff, the fragmentation of patient care and the dynamics of 'victimisation'. Smythe (1984, p. 227) explains this 'victimisation' as follows:

> Victim psychology is characterised by the concept that individuals in lower-status positions often tend to feel alienated from their peers. Rather than offering support and collectively defending their rights, they may pull against each other in backbiting or in open competition. This kind of horizontal violence is typical of low status groups who identify with the aggressor; members of low status groups are, at times, more critical and harsh towards their peers than are members of a high status group.

She then explains how this 'victimisation' process may apply to nurses:

> Nurses operating under high stress situations may be too survival-oriented to consider the needs of colleagues. Instead of having a reciprocal, supportive network of peers we develop pecking orders that only dole out stress to those lower in the hierarchy. (p. 228)

Developing and maintaining social support

Staff must first identify and take a risk by acknowledging their need for support to others. They must also identify the range of support needs that they have. Support needs are not just emotional, but also involve a variety of technical and practical issues. Buysen (1996) outlines in detail what this variety of support systems includes and how it can be developed.

Smythe (1984, pp. 232–3, 235–6) also suggests a variety of ways of developing such support networks both on and off the job:

Outside work
- Build support rituals and celebrations. Remember your birthday and other special events and share them with others.
- Extend your circle of friends and schedule regular get-togethers.
- Find others through interest groups and organisations not directly related to work.
- Seek to support others using the telephone or random acts of kindness, give to others in order to receive.
- Turn drudgery into celebrations with others.

At work
- Welcome new staff members through a comprehensive induction programme and buddy system.
- Spread the learning through mentors and appropriate supervision.
- Develop peer support groups at the workplace.

Such support can come from a wide range of sources beyond the immediate work group.

Sources of support

Often sources of support are seen in a fairly limited way; however, support can be gathered from a variety of sources as follows:

1. Self-support
2. Other workers/support group
3. Service users
4. Support person/consultant
5. Community
6. Other sources.

Let us now look at these sources of support.

Self-support strategies

Relaxation and self-management skills can be useful in coping with stress and trauma on the job. Smythe (1984) and Bailey (1985) offer some practical ideas in these areas.
These can include:

- Relaxation skills
- Time and self-management skills
- Continuing education and training
- Recording and reflecting.

Recording and reflecting on a situation of assault or trauma can include the following approaches:

1. Write down feelings quickly after a traumatic incident.
2. Later outline what were your desired outcomes for that situation.
3. Record what your actions were in the incident – how helpful were they in achieving your aims?
4. Attempt to summarise briefly all of the above.
5. Finally write down what needs to be done next.

The above process provides a structure within which workers can analyse their interactions and possible future actions in the light of the realities of the situation. This written format could also be shared with other workers.

There is an alternative to writing things down that involves placing thoughts, feelings and responses to an incident on audio-tape and then determining action similar to steps (4) and (5) above.

Other workers/support groups

This type of support can include:

- One-to-one support (emotional – co-counselling, defusing or technical support)
- Self-help groups (encouragement, practical help, stimulation through teaching – learning, problem-solving, practice)
- Forming task or working groups.

Task groups have two important support features for workers:

1. They provide an opportunity to meet with other workers with different experiences and ideas.
2. They give people time to concentrate on issues of particular concern to agree together how to present new ideas and strategies to an outside group.

Work groups need not focus only on the production of a specific piece of work (that is, occupational health and safety protocols or aggression management guidelines), but can also look at ways of improving a worker's general performance or satisfaction (that is, deciding on work priorities).

In setting up task groups, it is important that:

■ The task is clear
■ The time used is limited and specified
■ Someone takes responsibility for convening the meetings.

Health service users

It may not seem possible to consider service users as a source of support, but they are also concerned with their own and others' safety in health services and may, through patient groups, provide support for mutually beneficial change within the workplace.

Support person (internal)/consultant (external)

An internal support person could be a peer or a chosen supervisor concerned with the staff member's well-being. Such a person does not play a direct counselling role or that of a 'detective'.

Firth *et al.* (1987, p. 56) in their research, identified three distinctive aspects of positive personal support as displayed by the nurses' superiors:

These aspects appeared to coincide with those identified... as important to other helping relationships: personal respect or warmth; empathy, attention and listening skills; an absence of defensiveness.

Alongside an internal support person, an external consultant can provide:

- Stimulation (see possibilities, develop potential)
- Background knowledge
- Personal support (emotional)
- Practical support (ideas and skills)
- Security/buffer.

An external consultant should be someone trusted and respected by the worker who will challenge the health service worker to discover new approaches and take action towards increased effectiveness.

A consultant need not necessarily be involved in exactly the same work but have experience, skills and knowledge to make the necessary connections. His or her role is to help the worker become more expert through providing structured learning situations and acting as a sounding board.

Another approach is that of a small group consultancy. Here a small group of like-minded workers meet with a consultant who aims to help the participants to learn from each other and make progress in their work.

Community

Community-based support may be provided through professional bodies, interagency groups or patient action groups who wish to see the workplace a less violent situation for both patients and staff.

How to maintain support networks

Once support networks have been established, they must be carefully nurtured and maintained, and have the following characteristics:

- Be simple to establish and operate
- Be maintained easily
- Have equality/mutuality as their basis
- Be internally and externally based
- Have multiple sources
- Encourage feedback.

Adequate and effective support also needs to have direction and purpose through:

- stated and specific goals
- having structures for the support that encourages deeper exploration of the real issues and problems
- aiming for clarity through active listening, accurate feedback and summary
- being able to identify steps for actions.

If the aim and process are not clear, it is easy under work pressure to unintentionally destroy one's support system through misattribution, that is, blaming. Almost every time we see an event or behaviour, we try to find a cause for it. We can try to explain a person's response or behaviour towards us in two ways:

1. *Personality*. We blame the cause of an event upon another individual's personality.
2. *Situation*. We make situational explanations when we see the cause as arising from the situation.

People tend to explain their own actions in situational terms and the behaviour of others in personality terms. Thus when things go wrong for us on the job, we blame either our situation and/or the behaviour and personality of others.

In order to avoid sabotaging social support systems, it is essential for people periodically to reassess their earlier judgements of their friends, work colleagues and other contacts in order to avoid misjudging and misattributing. Avoid early judgements and give others the benefit of the doubt, and in this way you will avoid alienating your 'supporters'.

Sometimes this 'sabotage' occurs because we have not really identified what our support needs are and may not ask for them clearly and our potential supporters become confused or discouraged. So express your opinions and feelings clearly and tactfully, identify your and others' support needs.

So decide what you want, examine the implications of that decision (why do you want it?) and take a risk of not getting it, then ask for support and give it in return.

Following these guidelines should enable a worker to develop a strong and useful support network.

Agency responses to violence against health service workers

Preventive strategies

Naturally, any effective response to the issue of assaults against health service workers requires due consideration be given to the prevention of assaults as well as intervention after assaults have occurred. A number of preventive strategies are suggested by Brown *et al.* (1986), Bowie (1994, 1996), Bibby (1995) and others and are outlined below.

Staffing issues

- Sufficient and appropriate staff should be selected and employed.
- New staff should be given a full and appropriate induction into the work situation and the realistic risks involved.
- Staff should be given initial and ongoing training in the identification, prevention and reduction of violence.
- All staff should feel secure, supported and able to admit fears and negative emotions.
- Staff should be given anticipatory information on what constitutes normal worker reactions to stressful and abusive situations.
- Staff should feel confident in reporting violent incidents to their management and that such reports will be acted upon.
- The agency or organisation must provide clear practice and emergency guidelines for their staff if faced with actual or potential violence.

Staff management issues

Brown *et. al.* (1986) also suggest a number of specific agency responsibilities with regard to staff management, namely:

- To keep staff aware of the dangers of particular high-risk procedures, work situations and clients.
- To ensure that workers are not isolated and that help is always readily available.
- High-risk situations are allocated to those most able to cope with them.

- Appropriate back-up and support must be available to those working in community-based settings or patients' homes.
- Staff need to be made aware of the different approaches needed in working in a community- or home-based setting compared with an agency or in-patient setting.
- Good communication must be maintained between administration, staff and patients. Also good contacts must be maintained with police and emergency service personnel.
- All staff rosters and staffing combinations need to be worked out to reduce the risk to staff of confrontation or dangerous situations without curtailing the service.

Long-term issues

In the light of the sometimes long-term nature of assaulted staff's recuperation and the specialist services involved, good agency practice of long-term planning for preventive and support services should also include:

- The training of their own personnel where appropriate for the assessing, debriefing, counselling and referral of staff survivors of trauma
- Training their staff in the follow-up and support of staff survivors of trauma as peer supporters and defusers
- The use of outside agencies in the assessment of staff trauma and the provision of assistance and advice to co-workers in providing necessary understanding and support for staff survivors of trauma. Management should maintain good referral networks with external support agencies, both government and voluntary (for example, victim support schemes, legal and information services, unions and counselling services)
- The establishment of employee assistance committees.

Just who is to provide the longer-term support and possible therapeutic needs of assaulted staff members is open to debate. Some staff may not wish to be debriefed or counselled by members of their own organisation for a variety of valid reasons, including trust, confidentiality and career progression, while others may quite readily use 'in-house' services and resist contracted services. The related question of to what extent the use of post-trauma services should be mandatory or voluntary has been addressed in a variety of different ways by a range of health services.

In whatever way these services are to be provided to staff, there must be a comprehensive range of options from which staff can choose. Such services must also operate in a flexible way such that all staff, and not just the most vocal or knowledgeable, receive these services.

Administrators, managers and supervisors also need to be aware that organisational policies, structure and procedures may generate or alleviate situations leading to violence against workers. Greaves (1994, p. 225) emphasises this lack of organisational awareness or commitment:

> Despite being an organisational issue, violence at work appears to be one of the work related risks that employees are expected to cope with alone. Many employers have handed their responsibility for managing this health and safety problem to their employees. Focusing only on the employee is unlikely to provide a solution because this ignores the multitude of other factors involved.

An increasing focus must be upon the impact of organisational change and political forces in creating environments of staffing and resources shortages within the health services. Such changes are developing workplace environments of violence and aggression as the norm rather than the exception. No matter how professional the staff are, they cannot be held totally accountable for the violence-generating environment being created around them.

Moore (1993), Greaves (1994), Moore and Maguire (1995) and Cherry and Upton (1997) outline in detail the risk management and prevention strategies that organisations need to implement in a comprehensive approach to decreasing work-based violence.

Post-trauma agency support

Helping the staff survivors of trauma

As with others, 'helper' survivors of trauma may see themselves as weak, helpless, frightened and needy, and feel as if they have little control over their lives. They may need to mourn their loss of feelings of security and the related decreased sense of control and invulnerability, and to overcome a sense of being different from others.

Coping with the trauma of assault involves the worker coming to terms with the effect of these shattered world view assumptions and re-establishing a conceptual system that will allow him or her once again to function effectively. This process involves the re-establishment of a world view that can incorporate the worker's recent experience as a survivor of trauma without totally abandoning the previously held basic assumptions. These past assumptions need to be refashioned in order that they can also accommodate the worker's new experience. As previously indicated, this involves making sense of the event, restoring a sense of control, purpose and trust, and being able to plan for the future.

Thus, any successful resolution of a crisis situation involves dealing with loss and the related grief and bereavement, and helping the person to reconstruct shattered beliefs and regain some control over his or her life. This rebuilding and recovery involves the following issues:

■ Making sense of, or redefining, the event
■ Re-establishing a sense of control over one's life
■ Restoring a feeling of trust and self-worth
■ Re-establishing meaning, purpose and justice
■ Re-establishing balance and planning for the future.

The NOVA training programme (NOVA, undated) summarises these issues as the need to establish a climate of safety and security, ventilation and validation, and prediction and preparation.

Some intervention issues

As previously stated, health service survivors of trauma may be unwilling to accept the identity of victim or to seek any help, and may use established defences to block out, minimise or negate the event. However, such defences, or coping strategies, used during the event may be quite adaptive. Therapeutic endeavours that weaken or break down such defences can be extremely counter-productive. As Lenehan and Turner (1984) suggest, provided an individual's appraisal and defence strategies are assisting them to produce adaptive responses to the event and cope positively, a major intervention is probably not warranted.

There are currently few guidelines for distinguishing between helpful and unhelpful coping strategies that might be used by health service workers in responding to assaults against them. However, issues such as an individual's existing world view, available social support structures, and current work and life environment are obviously of considerable consequence in the development of such strategies.

An assumption here is that staff survivors of trauma are essentially psychologically healthy individuals facing a crisis. If evidence to the contrary is apparent, quite different, and perhaps more intensive, intervention strategies may be warranted.

Staff survivors of trauma have the same general difficulties in overcoming fear, anxiety, depression and phobic reactions as do other non-helper survivors of trauma. Hypervigilance, free-floating anxiety, irritability, repetitive intrusive thoughts and nightmares are common, as are feelings of helplessness and seeking a sense of safety and security. Anger invariably also appears in one form or another. However, it may be repressed or denied and appear as depression, or else be displaced on to others, including other patients/clients, staff members or significant others.

As has been noted with non-helper survivors of trauma, the strong emotions experienced immediately after an assault may be difficult to deal with. As a consequence, survivors of trauma may distance themselves from others who are trying to offer support, and may repress their emotional feelings and experience various psychosomatic symptoms. Intervention may also be needed with significant others in the staff member's life in order to help them understand their current state and support needs.

One way of meeting these needs is through the process called critical incident stress management.

Critical incident intervention and support

Support needs to be offered in a sensitive and aware fashion as soon as possible after the critical incident, that is, the violent act, so as not to induce secondary trauma. As in dealing with any assault victim, those initiating the intervention and support must be aware of their own emotions and possible projections on to staff survivors of trauma. Pity, condescension, distancing or blaming by supporters is damaging; instead, unqualified empathy and understanding in the context of peer and organisational support are crucial.

Rather than seeking individual counselling, the assaulted staff may need or want to discuss the incident and their reaction to it within the work situation and with fellow professionals and may choose not to see the assault as a personal attack. Thus if the worker wishes to deal with the assault within the work context and appears to be coping adequately, simple support is clearly sufficient intervention.

Early intervention within 24 hours can provide a solid basis for a more successful, more rapid resolution of the crisis situation. Staff survivors of trauma may first need help with immediate problem-solving and decision-making. This may include providing immediate first aid and medical help, dealing with emergency staff and police, completing medical and legal reports, and providing transport and companionship at home.

At the same time, the staff should have immediate extensive opportunities to talk about their feelings about the assault with their colleagues and superiors. Debriefing in a non-blaming fashion should be available and provided in a manner that develops the skills for handling future incidents.

Mitchell (1984, Mitchell and Everly 1993) has developed a comprehensive model for doing the above which he calls Critical Incident Stress Debriefing (CISD) to minimise the negative impact of crisis situations on helpers. The CISD concept is a developing one, with a potential application to assaulted health service workers.

CISD is a psychological and educational group process designed especially for workers, with two purposes in mind. First, CISD is designed to mitigate the impact of critical incidents on the person. Second, CISD is designed to accelerate normal recovery in normal people who are experiencing the normal signs, symptoms and reactions to totally abnormal events.

CISD team leaders should not be supervisors with direct managerial responsibility for the staff being debriefed.

Mitchell and Everly (1993, p. 128) explain the key concepts behind debriefing and defusing as follows:

1. Early intervention
2. Opportunity for catharsis
3. Opportunity to verbally reconstruct the trauma
4. Establishment of a behavioural structure within which to conduct the group process (a behavioural 'road map' of sorts)
5. Establishment of a structured psychological progression (a psychological 'road map' of sorts)
6. Group support

7. Peer support
8. Opportunity for follow-up.

The CISD process has a number of steps, as outlined below.

Introduction
The introduction serves to introduce members of the CISD team and present some ground rules. It is emphasised that confidentiality is paramount and that CISD is neither therapy nor an investigation of the event.

Fact phase
Here the events, as they unfold for the workers, are recounted from their individual perspectives.

Thought phase
Here workers are asked to describe the most prominent thought or thoughts that filled their minds at the time of the trauma.

Reaction phase
In this phase, workers are asked what was the worst or most disturbing aspect of this event for them.

Symptom phase
Here workers are asked to describe any cognitive, emotional, physical or behavioural reactions they may have experienced during or since the traumatic incident.

Teaching phase
During this phase, the normality and variety of human responses to trauma are outlined, as are strategies for handling future reactions and setting goals for eventual 'recovery'.

Re-entry phase
Here the process is drawn to a close, the participants affirmed and ongoing support offered if necessary.

A supportive approach, rather than a therapeutic one, can set the tone for the initial intervention as one of developing mastery and strength without down-playing the extreme trauma experienced. There is a danger that, in conveying an expectation of a deep, reactive emotional trauma, a self-fulfilling prophesy may be created.

However, staff should be given information about their own possible responses and feelings as survivors, and the acceptability and naturalness of such reactions. It is stressed that their reactions are those of normal people reacting normally to an abnormal event. Some care must be exercised in using the CISD approach in the health services. It was initially developed in an emergency services context and may not be directly applied without some sensitive modification to the new context. This approach may not be effective when used with multidisciplinary health teams as the 'established pecking order' in the team may stop open sharing of trauma experiences.

In the light of the possible danger of secondary trauma being inflicted upon staff survivors by colleagues through blaming, distancing, hesitancy or overly emotional reactions, a high level of co-worker awareness and sensitivity needs to be encouraged and maintained.

Mitchell, in his article 'Teaming up against critical incident stress' (1986, p. 26), suggests that these problems can be overcome in part by training workers as 'peer counsellors'. He describes peer counsellors as staff members who are trained to provide the first basic support to their traumatised fellow workers. He refers to part of this support process as defusing. Peer counsellors are often the ones who let management know that a structured debriefing may be required. Peer defusers are usually present in CISD group sessions. Mitchell and Everly (1993) and Tunnecliffe and Roy (1993) give more details about the process of training peer defusers. Environmental barriers such as agency or staff indifference to the problem may also make trauma support by co-workers difficult.

A small number of staff will need long-term, more therapeutic interventions, especially if showing symptoms of post-traumatic stress disorder. Flannery (1992) and Hodgkinson and Stewart (1991) outline in more detail some of the therapeutic options available for deeply traumatised staff.

One recent supportive and apparently more therapeutic approach is that of Eye Movement Desensitisation and Reprocessing (EMDR). This approach seems to have some similarities with behavioural flooding. It is believed that the brain's ability to process information breaks down under extreme trauma, the distressing information becoming 'frozen' in the memory and not resolved. EMDR attempts to identify this unprocessed traumatic information and free it up so it can be properly resolved and the impact of the event greatly diminished. This release comes through the use of rapid eye movement in the client induced by the therapist. Although highly experimental at present, EMDR seems to be achieving substantial if not sometimes controversial results. This approach is described in more detail in Hodgkinson and Stewart (1991).

Such personal support strategies also need to be seen in the context of broader responses that the employer's agency needs to be able to implement. If this does not occur, the 'blame' for the incident or the responsibility for its resolution will continue to be laid at the feet of the workers.

Agency responsibilities

To minimise the negative consequences of assaults and violence when they do occur, and to provide optimal assistance to staff survivors of trauma, some specific guidelines for agency action can be suggested:

- Staff should have immediate opportunities to talk about their feelings surrounding the assault with colleagues and administrators. Mitchell refers to this process as a defusing.
- If necessary, a more structured debriefing in a non-blaming fashion should be available within 24 hours. It should be provided in a manner that develops the worker's skills for handling future incidents.
- Staff should be given information about their own possible responses and feelings as survivors of trauma and the acceptability and naturalness of such reactions.
- Practical help and support should be made available, including offers of ongoing personal protection, a carefully supervised or changed workload or the possibility of job sharing.
- Allowing time off from the job or time out in an alternative work location could be another practical response. Help regarding training and seeking other career opportunities may also be needed.
- The associates, administrators, co-workers, friends and family of the staff survivors of trauma should be made aware of the worker's possible feelings, responses and needs, and wherever necessary be helped in their support for the assaulted person. These associates, and the agency, need to remain aware of the long-term nature of the recovery from violence and its trauma.

Often, more than short-term crisis intervention is needed, and intervention might need to involve the rebuilding of the survivor of trauma's assumptive world. For example, the possible effects of the assault on changing the staff survivor's view of the patient/client and the agency may also need to be recognised and dealt with.

■ In order that staff are not further stigmatised for seeking trauma counselling or taking part in violence prevention programmes, these programmes should be part of a broader continuing education aspect of an organisation's training.

This broader approach could include topics such as induction to the organisation, preventive stress management programmes, communication and assertion skills, group and leadership skills, and healthy lifestyle information.

Assistance programmes for staff survivors of trauma

Potential barriers to programmes

Engels and Marsh (1986) point out that many forces work against the acceptance of an employee assistance programme by both management and workers.

Many professional helping staff have difficulty seeing themselves as, or accepting the role of, a victim. In addition, since violence is perpetrated by those in their care, staff often do not accept assault as a work-related accident but instead view it as part of the conditions of the job. Thus this view excuses the behaviour of the patient or client and is often further condoned by the agency through its silence or inaction.

The *milieu* of the tight-knit, helping community also often makes it difficult for workers to express feelings of fear or uncertainty about their clients and the work situation. This, in turn, makes it hard for individuals or work teams to accept or actively support assaulted staff assistance schemes for themselves.

Unless an injury makes it difficult for staff members to stay at work, they often continue on the job trying to minimise the abuse faced until stress and low morale take their toll. Thus assaulted workers are often left isolated from their peers, feeling apathetic and angry, and trying to withdraw.

A third negative force against accepting such schemes is the previously mentioned blaming and distancing attitude displayed by co-workers. For other workers to admit to the necessity for such assistance programmes for others, let alone themselves, once again challenges the workers' feelings of invulnerability.

In the light of such potential resistance by staff to such programmes, they should be presented as part of an overall staff education and preventive health programme, as previously mentioned. By including aggression management skills among such topics, workers are given preventive information and are not stigmatised for attending such courses. Also, in this way, the question of violence in the workplace is not sensationalised, and the unnecessary arousing of staff anxiety is avoided.

Bailey (1985) outlines a personal and organisational support system for nurses and other medical personnel to combat stress. At the personal level, he considers in detail five methods of stress control: progressive relaxation, relaxation with desensitisation, transcendental meditation, autogenic regulation training and stress inoculation training. He then goes on to stress the importance of also taking into account the effects of the workers' organisation in promoting or diminishing their physical and emotional well-being:

> However much more requires to be done by the organisations of the health care system to care for those charged with the awesome responsibility of providing care. In a nutshell, there must be more new and radical ways of providing care for care givers. I am persuaded the way ahead here is to set up counselling and consultation services for health professionals to help them better cope with the demands of caring. (pp. 136–7)

He believes that such a service should deal not only with post-trauma care and support, but also the preventive aspects:

> In practical terms, health consultation services combining restorative and preventative facilities to aid health professionals coping are desirable. (p. 139)

This could serve as a model, with some modifications, for the above-suggested aggression trauma management programmes, as part of a continuing education format. Such a support system could undertake many of the functions outlined above.

However, despite such barriers, successful employee assistance programmes for victims of violence have been implemented and can serve as useful models. Some programmes for armed hold-up and bank robbery victims also have much to teach those initiating such services in the health, welfare and community service sectors.

Obviously, such comprehensive programmes may be more easily sponsored by large medical and welfare organisations. Smaller services may need greater access to outside counselling and support services in a flexible way in order to meet the needs of their own staff.

Implementing assistance programmes

In the light of the above, and having regard for the particular needs and responses of staff survivors of trauma, an employee assistance programme should include a number of different services. These may encompass medical attention, trauma support and counselling, legal advice, and information on compensation, workers' rights and other health and safety issues.

Engels and Marsh (1986) suggest the formation of a permanent committee in each agency to oversee such programmes and guarantee the rights of both clients and employees. Such committees would be similar to those already functioning in some health care establishments in the United Kingdom, Canada and Australia under occupational Health and Safety legislation.

They suggest that the role and tasks of such committees should comprise:

■ The creation and monitoring of an on-call team to deal with violent incidents
■ Making sure that guidelines and procedures for dealing with violent clients and employee traumas are formulated and carried out
■ The collection of incident reports and the collation of appropriate strategies
■ The careful examination of each violent episode, with appropriate recommendations about future action and an evaluation of their outcomes.

These committee responsibilities as outlined by Engels and Marsh are only some of the wide-ranging aspects involved in the implementation of such employee assistance programmes.

Dawson *et al.* (1998) describe a structured response team to provide support for assaulted staff members. Their Assault Support Team (AST) aimed to provide emotional support and resolution of role conflict for assaulted staff. AST team members were required to attend training that focused on the dynamics of assault, common responses of assaulted staff and how to provide supportive interventions. The AST programme operates on a 'buddy' team approach whereby therapeutic staff are paired and given the role of providing intervention for members of other teams in the facility. The effectiveness of the AST approach is difficult to ascertain, but it did seem to have some effect on decreasing staff turnover.

A somewhat similar but more comprehensive approach, the Assaulted Staff Action Program (ASAP), is described by Flannery *et al.* (1991). It has three levels: first that of front-line staff on call to provide defusing to colleagues on their shift; next, supervisors who provide back-up for defusers, track the needs of assaulted staff and assess ongoing training needs; and third, the ASAP director who monitors the quality of the ASAP programme and provides supervision and in-service training for staff as well as a weekly support group for assaulted staff and a hospital-wide stress management group.

This seems a promising approach to the post-trauma management of staff assault at an organisational and team level.

Conclusion

It is unlikely that violent assaults against health service workers can be eliminated, especially in a context of apparently increasing levels of violent behaviour in the general community.

It is imperative, however, that helping professionals attempt to overcome their illusions of invulnerability and make themselves aware of this issue and its relevance for both themselves and their colleagues. Thus they can assist their various employers to develop and implement strategies that will hopefully minimise both the incidence of the problem and its damaging consequences to individual helpers.

However, the onus for taking appropriate action should not lie just with the individual workers. An equally heavy responsibility lies with the health service organisations and their managements to take the major initiatives in violence prevention, management and post-trauma support. Without such initiatives, responses by individuals are likely to be partial and fragmented and thus ineffectual.

References

Bailey R. (1985) *Coping with Stress in Caring*, Netherlands B.V., Blackwell Scientific.

Bibby P. (1995) *Personal Safety for Health Care Workers*, Ashgate, Arena.

Bowie V. (1994) *Violence in the Workplace*. Submission to the Industry Commission Inquiry into Occupational Health and Safety, Sydney, October.

Bowie V. (1996) *Coping with Violence: A Guide for the Human Services*, London, Whitting & Birch.

Brown R., Bute S. and Ford P. (1986) *Social Workers at Risk*, Basingstoke, Macmillan.

Buysen H. (1996) *Traumatic Experiences of Nurses: When Your Profession Becomes a Nightmare*, London, Jessica Kingsley.

Cherry D. and Upton B. (1997) *Managing Potentially Violent Situations: A Guide for Workers and Organisations*. Melbourne, Centre for Social Health.

Dawson J., Johnston M., Kehiayan N et al. (1988) Response to patient assault, *Psychosocial Nursing and Mental Health*, February: 8–11, 15.

Duffy E. (1995) Horizontal violence: a conundrum for nursing, *Collegian*, 2(2): 5–17.

Engels F. and Marsh S. (1986) Helping the employee victim of violence in hospitals, *Hospital and Community Psychiatry*, 37(2): 159–62.

Farrell G. (1997) Aggression in clinical settings: nurses views, *Journal of Advanced Nursing*, 25: 501–8.

Firth H., McKeown P., McIntee J. et al. (1987) Burnout, personality and support in long stay nursing, *Nursing Times*, 83(32): 55–7.

Flannery R. (1992) *Post-traumatic Stress Disorder: The Victim's Guide to Healing and Recovery*, New York, Crossroad.

Flannery R., Fulton P., Tausch J. et al. (1991) A programme to help staff cope with the psychological sequelae of assaults by patients, *Hospital and Community Psychiatry*, 42: 935–8.

Greaves A. (1994) Organisational approaches to the prevention and management of violence. In Whykes T. and Mezey G. (eds) *Violence and Health Professionals*, London, Chapman & Hall.

Hodgkinson P. and Stewart M. (1991) *Coping with Catastrophe: A Handbook of Disaster Management*, London, Routledge.

Jannoff-Bulman R. (1985) The aftermath of victimisation: re-building shattered assumptions, in Figley C. (ed.) *Trauma and its Wake*, New York, Brunner/Mazel.

Jannoff-Bulman R. (1992) *Shattered Assumptions: Towards a New Psychology of Trauma*, New York, Macmillan.

Jannoff-Bulman R., Madden M. and Timko C. (1983) Victims reaction to aid: the role of perceived vulnerability. In Nadler A., Fisher J. and DePaulo B.M. (eds) *New Directions in Helping*, vol. 3, New York, Academic Press.

Kahn A.S. (1984) *Victims of Crime and Violence: Final Report of the APA Task Force on the Victims of Crime and Violence.* Washington, DC, American Psychological Association.

Kahn J. and Earle E. (1982) *The Cry for Help and the Professional Response,* Oxford, Pergamon Press.

Lanza M. (1983) The reactions of nursing staff to physical assault by a patient, *Hospital and Community Psychiatry,* **34**(1): 44–7.

Lanza M. (1987) The relationship of the severity of assault to blame placement for assault, *Archives of Psychiatric Nursing,* **4**: 269–79.

Lenehan G.P. and Turner J. (1984) Treatment of staff victims of violence. In Turner J. (ed.) *Violence in a Medical Care Setting: A Survival Guide,* Maryland, Aspen.

Lerner M. (1980) *The Belief in a Just World: A Fundamental Delusion,* New York, Plenum Press.

Levy B. and Brown V. (1984) Strategies for crisis intervention with victims of violence. In Saunders S. (ed.) *Violent Individuals and Families,* Springfield, IL, Charles C. Thomas.

Mitchell J. (1983) When disaster strikes: a critical incident debriefing process, *Journal of Emergency Medical Services,* **8**(1): 36–9.

Mitchell J.T. (1984) No time for goodbyes, *JEMS,* September: 28–30.

Mitchell J.T. (1986) Teaming up against critical incident stress, *Chief Fire Executive,* **84**: 24–6.

Mitchell J. and Everly G. (1993) *Critical Incident Stress Debriefing: An Operations Manual for the Prevention of Traumatic Stress Among Emergency Services and Disaster Workers,* Maryland, Chevron.

Mitchell J.T. and Resnik H.L.P. (1981) *Emergency Response to Crisis.* Englewood Cliffs, NJ, Prentice-Hall.

Moore W. (1993) *Ensuring Staff Safety: How to Audit the Risk from Attack at Work,* Birmingham, Pepar.

Moore W. and Maguire J. (1995) *Handling Aggression and Violence in Health Services.* Birmingham, Pepar.

National Organisation for Victim Assistance (NOVA) (Undated) *Crisis and Stress,* Washington, DC, NOVA.

Peterson C. and Seligman M. (1983) Learned helplessness and victimisation, *Journal of Social Issues,* **39**(2): 103–16.

Pines A., Aronson E. and Kafry D. (1981) *Burnout: From Tedium to Personal Growth,* New York, Free Press.

Ravenscroft T. (1994) After the crisis, *Nursing Times,* **90**(12): 26–8.

Rowett C. (1986) *Violence in Social Work,* Cambridge, University of Cambridge Institute of Criminology.

Ryan J. and Poster E. (1989) The assaulted nurse: short-term and long-term responses, *Archives of Psychiatric Nursing,* **3**(6): 323–31.

Smythe E. (1984) *Surviving Nursing,* New York, Addison-Wesley.

Tunnecliffe M. and Roy O. (1993) *Emergency Support: A Handbook for Peer Supporters,* Western Australia, Bayside Books.

Whykes T. and Whittington R. (1994) Reactions to assault. In Whykes T. and Mezey G. (eds) *Violence and Health Care Professionals,* London, Chapman & Hall.

9

A SYSTEM OF EDUCATION AND TRAINING FOR THE CARE AND MANAGEMENT OF PEOPLE WITH SPECIAL NEEDS WHO DISPLAY VIOLENT OR DANGEROUS BEHAVIOURS

Colin Beacock

Introduction

The provision of effective therapeutic nursing care within a multi-disciplinary context, for people with mental health problems and/or learning disabilities who may present with dangerous criminal and/or violent propensities, requires a skilled and specialist nursing staff. The need for education specific to this area of practice has been apparent from at least 1971 (Department of Health and Social Security) when the *Revised Report of the Working Party on Security in Psychiatric Hospitals* (Glancy Report) noted that the lack of appropriate educational opportunities was hindering attempts to improve quality of care. This observation was echoed more recently in the Reed Report (Department of Health and Home Office 1992), which suggested that inadequate educational provision at specialist level continued to be a problem. This sentiment found support in the conclusions of NE Thames and SE Thames RHAs (1994) *Report of the Inquiry into the Care and Treatment of Christopher Clunis* (Clunis Report), which stated that:

The assessment of the risk of violence should never be a hasty guess following a simple examination of the patient's current mental state at interview. It is a skill to be learned and refreshed from time to time by anyone who has responsibility to respond to the needs of people showing disturbed behaviour. Psychiatrists and other mental health workers need to be trained in this skill as do, at the appropriate level, general practitioners and other members of the primary health care team, social workers, police and probation officers. At the very least they should be given sufficient training to recognise the limits of their personal knowledge and to understand the role of forensic services. (p. 119)

In highlighting a scientific approach to the assessment of risk, based upon multiagency and interdisciplinary programmes of education and training, the Report illustrates some of the fundamental principles that should guide and inform educational programmes, designed to prepare the person who will work with those who may have a propensity to display violent and aggressive behaviour.

The Report investigated the care and treatment of a man whose mental health had deteriorated to the extent that his potential for violence was well recognised by a series of health and social care workers. Where they failed was in constructing a system and process by which the recognition of Christopher Clunis's needs could be communicated, translated and acted upon by a range of service providers. The death of Jonathan Zito was a tragedy for both himself and his killer Christopher Clunis. It was, in all probability, avoidable. It is now evident that an educational programme, preparing staff to work co-operatively in the care of violent and aggressive people, could have significantly decreased the likelihood of Christopher Clunis attacking a stranger and enabled him to enjoy a more rewarding social role.

The Clunis Report's recommendations are echoed in a number of the inquiries summarised by Sheppard's (1994) review of mental health inquiry reports published in England and Wales. Recommendations for improving practice need to be considered within the context of the contemporary educational systems that prepare workers to meet their responsibilities in respect of this challenging client group. Currently, formal recognition via the statutory bodies governing the education of nurse practitioners working in this field of care is offered by the respective national boards – the English National Board (ENB), the National Board for Nursing, Midwifery and Health Visiting for Scotland (NBS), the Welsh National Board (WNB) and the Northern Ireland National Board (NINB) – which have delegated responsibility from the United Kingdom Central

Council for Nursing, Midwifery and Health Visiting (UKCC) to accredit basic and post-basic courses in respect of the training and education of nurses. The ENB has formulated guidelines that indicate a need to offer opportunities for pre-registration nursing students to have formal training in the management of violence and aggression, focusing primarily upon personal protection. They have also formulated an outline curriculum for the accreditation of post-basic courses that equip nursing staff with the skills and knowledge to manage manifestations of violence and aggression. The ENB guidelines may be criticised, however, for lacking compulsion, offering only a potential framework for course design, with indicative content. While promoting innovation in curriculum development, it may also lead to a piecemeal approach with no regulation of minimum standards and produce a uniprofessional approach to care management. This is arguably more likely to promote, rather than prevent, incidents such as the case of Christopher Clunis.

In Scotland, the NBS have recently validated the first Specialist Practitioner Programme in Forensic Psychiatric Nursing in the United Kingdom under the Council's Standards for Education and Practice Following Registration, more usually known as PREPP (UKCC 1994). In addition, a number of programmes offering an academically validated award, either alone or in combination with professional development, also exist, including programmes offered by the University of Manchester, the University of Stirling (via distance learning) and the University of Dundee.

It appears that after long neglect this area of practice has become the focus of some potentially important educational initiatives. What is of importance, however, is that such innovations reflect the unique needs of this area of practice together with changing ideas on the nature and purpose of education.

Defining and describing educational outcomes

Traditional approaches to curriculum design implore the curriculum planner to examine the philosophical basis that the course will reflect. To a large degree, this is a reflection of humanistic approaches to course design that have their roots in principles of self-actualisation and learner-centred approaches. While this chapter recognises the value of such debate and in no way wishes to denigrate the humanistic approach, the proposed model for curriculum design is deliberately simple and focuses upon the needs of the client and the attendant practice skills of the care staff as the basis upon which to develop the course content and assessment method. The argument will be established that it is the organisational philosophy that establishes, enables or limits the potential of the educational process, and that this should be the starting point for curriculum planning.

The model proposed derives from earlier work by the author in respect of educational methods and their application in areas of secure forensic care. The following model for curriculum design (Figure 9.1) is offered.

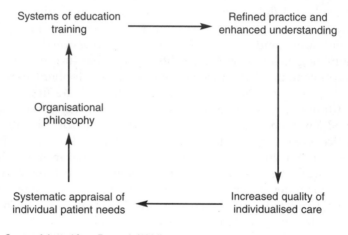

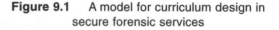

Source: Adapted from Beacock (1994).

Figure 9.1   A model for curriculum design in secure forensic services

Within this model, the emphasis is on the application in practice of refined skills and enhanced knowledge, arising out of an educational programme that is derived from a particular understanding of individual patient needs and potentials. The model allows for assessment methods that are sufficiently flexible to befit any stage of the learning cycle. A student can, therefore, be assessed in a variety of settings and at any stage of the learning cycle: in either the theoretical or practice setting within the educational programme, in the practice and application of refined and enhanced skills and knowledge; in the measurement of the quality of service provision, based upon individualised or group approaches; or through the analysis of the developmental needs of individual patients within the care planning process. Equally, the philosophy of an organisation can be assessed in terms of its relevance in practice.

A further consideration of each of these points will be developed, but an insight into how these applications of an assessment method might be guided by principles of a particular form of education is offered by Tuxworth (1989), who describes Competence Based Education and Training (CBET). He proposes that adopting CBET does not diminish the importance of knowledge and understanding but does, however, change the rationale for its incorporation into the curriculum, where its role becomes more explicitly to underpin practice competence. Methods of occupational/professional analysis should be sophisticated enough to give a multidimensional view of competence, and CBET has great potential in continuing professional development, particularly where it is necessary to ensure that professionals maintain and adapt their competencies to new conditions. Licensed occupations need to maintain competence through continuing professional development and regular performance review. The notion of 'minimum competence levels' is useful for certification purposes but carries some risks if these are the only standards available.

Minimum standards have been set by UKCC for maintaining an effective registration for all nurses (UKCC 1994) via PREPP, which requires all nurses wishing to maintain an entry on the register to demonstrate compliance via the creation and maintenance of a portfolio indicating ongoing professional development. The issue of competence has clear ramifications outside nursing, with all professions and organisations depending on high-level performance for their success. Acceptance of this premise leads on to consideration of multidisciplinary education.

The context of multidisciplinary education and training

The care of people whose needs challenge the resources of service providers is viewed as being at the margins of both health and social care services. Many of the client group find themselves in a position of being ill defined by the terms of legislation and social policy. For the purposes of this chapter, the group concerned is taken to be those people who are described by the Mental Health Act 1983 and Mental Health (Scotland) Act 1984 as having a 'mental disorder' or 'mental impairment or severe mental impairment', and those described by the Mental Health Act 1983 as having a 'personality disorder'. As is illustrated by the case of Christopher Clunis, such individuals are, over time, likely to find themselves receiving services in a number of settings, from a number of agencies, ranging from non-residential community services, through local and regional mental health services with varying levels of security, to prisons and young offenders' institutions.

Thus co-operation between services is required in practice and by policy. Many of the patients in this client group are subject to care programming initiatives and the supervision order provisions of the Mental Health Patients in the Community Bill. The divide between health and social care need is, therefore, arguably, increasingly being rendered redundant. What presents is an opportunity to structure systems of education and training that cross professional and health/social care boundaries but which are specific in their application to client needs. This would emerge as a form of multidisciplinary educational programme with accreditation from a number of different professional agencies and academic and/or vocational bodies, as has emerged in services for people with learning disabilities over recent years. A review of joint and shared learning initiatives in this area of practice was undertaken by Brown (1994), who described the context and significance of these approaches when he stated that 'Multi-disciplinary training is being actively promoted by central government' (p. 63). This emphasis on shared education has featured in several White Papers in the late 1980s and also in documents with a more specific focus. For example, the Tomlinson Report, published at the end of 1992, on health services in London, advocated multidisciplinary training for medical practitioners at both undergraduate and post-graduate levels (Tomlinson 1992).

The multidisciplinary 'mix' highlights issues of demarcation between occupational groups that shared learning explicitly recognises. At the same time, shared learning can begin to 'blur' boundaries in such a way that parallels the arguments for a seamless service (Audit Commission 1986). If contemporary arguments for developing services assume that traditional professional and service boundaries are no longer appropriate, shared learning represents a potential vehicle for re-examining and redefining those boundaries.

A system of education and training with plural accreditations and which capitalises on both academic and vocational assessment methodologies has the opportunity to develop a strong contemporary value. Where the curriculum development that underpins it is sufficiently flexible to ensure that a course keeps pace with contemporary issues and the social/political/economic features of the day, a programme that prepares the multiagency team to effectively manage potential manifestations of violence and aggression, and the appropriate delivery of services for this client group, could have significant credibility.

Enacting the curriculum model

In considering the process of education and training, it is essential that one commences with the recognition that it is the services to the client group which are central to that whole process. For that reason, although the model presented is cyclical, it would appear appropriate to commence by examining that particular aspect of the cycle that focuses upon specific client needs.

Systematic appraisal of individual patient needs

In the title of this section lies one of the prime dilemmas of the learning cycle. The idea of 'service users' being described as 'patients' is anathema to many of the care workers who provide services for this client group. What the title illustrates, therefore, are a number of features associated with the systems of care offered.

First, there is the issue of industrial language. It could be suggested that the verbal descriptors used when referring to the client group are indicative of the values base of the care workers who use them and that 'labelling' of the client group is prejudicial and stigmatising. At the same time, this offers immense opportunity for debate, analysis and theorising within systems of education and training. Whereas this may appear as a tension between different professional groups, it is the very nature of that tension that enables the group to flourish within the learning cycle.

Second, the title insists that the individualisation of systems of care is a prerequisite for the learning cycle. This indicates a need for philosophies to be enacted in practice rather than appearing as statements of guidance or intent.

Third, the fact that certain members of the client group are 'patients' supports the concept of life-long planning for the needs of the individual. That a person who has some form of learning disability, mental illness or social impairment might become a patient within the context of contemporary services would appear to be unquestionable. The debate surrounding the appropriateness of this situation is, once again, the very matter upon which the educational programme should be built.

It is usual for curriculum documents to commence with a statement of educational philosophy. There may be some considerable discrepancy in the effects of that educational philosophy in that it might influence theoretical aspects of the educational programme without ever finding application in the service areas of the organisation. At the same time, the espoused statements of the organisation may well have no relevance to the circumstances in which individual clients finds themselves. Goffman (1961) describes this phenomenon and considers that it illustrates the divide between idealism and reality in institutional care. This is a recurrent theme in forensic services, but it is nonetheless the ability, or lack of it, of service philosophies to impinge upon and inform the practices and activities of the care system that is of prime relevance to the client.

In seeking to substantiate this concept, it is from the field of services for people with learning disabilities that an explanation emerges. The Department of Health (1993) examined the needs of people with what have been described as 'challenging behaviours', many of whom might at some time during their development appear to be violent and aggressive individuals. Their report concluded that (Department of Health 1993, p. 65)

Whatever the situation for which staff are being recruited the demands on them are likely to flow from the programme of care and treatment which it is intended to adopt. It needs to be acknowledged from the outset that working with people with a learning disability can make heavy demands upon staff, but work with people with special needs can be even more demanding. Staff working with this client group should know from the start what will be expected of them, and should have a clear idea of the programme of the particular establishment in which they are working and of the overall service.

That is to say, the more sophisticated and challenging the system of care, the more will be the demands placed upon the care staff. Wherever they function, these staff must be aware of the values and philosophy of the service because that is what drives the programmes of care and treatment being offered. In consequence, where a person with a mental disorder and problems of violent or aggressive behaviour may historically have been effectively simply incarcerated, the care staff may have been generally obliged to do nothing more than act as custodians. No matter how sophisticated or libertarian the educational philosophy of the organisation for which they work, the informal culture of the organisation may reflect its origins rather more than its current role, and it may exert a powerful influence on the educational process. In such circumstances, the 'operational' philosophy is dictated by the informal rather than the formal systems of the organisation. To establish a curriculum based upon any premise other than this reality would lead to failure in that it would not influence or affect the quality of care received by the individual client or service user. What is essential is that the client group considered within this paper are viewed as people with 'special needs' rather than as current or potential criminals.

It is from this perspective that the 'systematic appraisal of individual patient needs' should be considered. Before commencing a programme of education and training, it is essential that the organisation as a whole, and the practice base of the outcoming student in particular, is in a position to accept the need for continuous development of competence in practice. It would not be sufficient for an organisation to demonstrate that it had formalised structures that governed multidisciplinary assessment. Instead, they would need to demonstrate how these needs assessments were utilised to assist in the prioritising of service developments. This would require some form of action planning for quality that involved 'consumers' in the broadest sense, for example clients, workers, relatives and purchasers. From an analysis of individual needs, a programme of education and training that reflected the reality of service delivery and consumption could be developed. Curriculum design and development would be a further extension of this process and its monitoring would provide a valuable adjunct to the quality monitoring systems of the organisation.

This concept need not emerge from an élitist base. Where an organisation aspires to achieve this form of service and has the commitment to pursue it, it has the potential to provide such programmes. Within the context of multiagency and multidisciplinary systems of service delivery, it is far more likely that the base unit for developing the course might be an amalgam of interested parties who each share ambitions and can 'own' a common philosophy.

Systems of education and training

If the operational philosophy of the organisation as a whole dictates the methodology of curriculum planning, it is enacted through the programmes of education and training that prepare the student to work, at whatever level, with the violent or aggressive person. Much formal educational activity in this area has focused upon direct physical interventions with clients who are displaying violence and/or aggression (Department of Health and Special Hospitals Authority 1992). While this has met the requirements of most organisations in the health and social care sectors, it may well reflect the way in which the operational philosophies of these organisations affect client care. It is clear that the priority of the organisations in question is to provide a safe and secure workplace for staff and residents. What is not evident is how these organisations intend to develop and refine their services to provide developmental opportunities for individual clients without an extension in this training input. Any extension would need to involve the challenging of practitioners and care workers so that they could recognise how the needs of individual clients were being met through interventions other than control and restraint methods. It is not sufficient to simply send staff on 'refresher' or 'update' training in control and restraint techniques. This would only measure their minimum level of competence.

Any system of education and training would need to be based upon a recognition of the genesis of violent and aggressive behaviours and an understanding of the physical, societal and psychological features associated with this phenomenon. The level of understanding of the particular student may well be dictated by his or her role within the organisation. The student's ability to recognise, however, that individualised needs assessment and care planning are transferable across agencies may need to be a prominent theme in course work.

The current situation is such that many services for this client group are provided within the context of non-specific psychiatric or social services departments. What is being proposed is an educational system that would support the views and proposals of successive reports (Department of Health and Social Security 1971, Department of Health and Social Security and Home Office 1974, Royal College of Psychiatrists 1980, Department of Health and Special Hospitals Authority 1992) and that addresses the attendant deficiencies in services as identified within the NE and SE Thames RHA Report (1994).

For this reason, there would need to be recognition that service organisation and structure would dictate the enactment of theory in practice, and that the value of education and training inputs should recognise not only the operational philosophy of the organisation as their baseline, but also the level of specificity of service to the client group within the organisation. It is within the context of developing a service that offers a degree of specialism in the management of people whose care needs are complicated by their violent and/or aggressive behaviours that the content of systems of education and training should evolve.

Many of the techniques and methods of management and intervention that are appropriate and desirable with this client group do not have value in other areas of care. At the same time, techniques and methods will be primarily drawn from the mainstream systems of practice. This is not to suggest that programmes of education and training should be based upon techniques that are exclusive to this client group but that it is very often the intensity of application which may vary, depending upon the specific needs of individual clients. While some content within the programme of education and training may have application in other circumstances and at other stages of the client's life plan, there is a progressional factor in the level of application which must be closely monitored. In much the same way that the client must be viewed as having 'special needs', services must be seen as being progressional in application and sufficiently flexible to change with the needs of the client.

Violent and aggressive behaviours are not uncommon in those people who have been described as constituting the client group, any more than they are not uncommon in any member of society. One of the problems with the teaching of interventions such as control and restraint techniques is that they tend to be given universal application within the service. If the proposed model of curriculum design is to function, it is essential that it is seen within the context of discreet and intensive therapeutic services that are designed to promote the habilitation or rehabilitation of the client. The degree of input that each student brings to the care programme of individual clients will vary with their role. What is an essential prerequisite is that students function with a discreet and identified individual or group of clients. In much the same way that referrals of clients to services need to be well justified, so the criteria for the selection of students to undertake programmes of education and training must be determined by their acceptance and recognition of the duty of care that is inherent in providing for this client group. It is from this principle that the content of the educational system must emanate.

While there may be some justification for offering developmental programmes for care staff across a broader range of service provision, it should be within the context of attempting to provide a 'seamless service'. Moreover, the content, while promoting cross-agency dialogue and care planning, must recognise the level of intensity of application required within the staff's role and service environment.

The content of the programmes of education and training would need to reflect service specificity. Whereas an understanding of risk assessment is essential for all care workers, the application in practice would vary between individuals depending upon their role and the level of needs of the individual client. What would be essential is that the outcomes of the process of education are evaluated through their interpretation in practice. The assessment method should be such that academic appraisal is geared to action research and the evaluation of impacts brought about through interventions and interactions with consumers and clients. In the same manner, practice skills should afford the appraisal of how they are adapted and developed in the light of changing circumstances and client need. Practice placements should reflect this principle and afford the individual opportunity to rehearse their skills in a variety of settings with a range of clients with varying levels of need. If the concept of relating curriculum development to quality enhancement, as previously described, is applied, the course content will develop in such a way that levels of application will emerge that are commensurate with the range and type of services provided.

The specific content of programmes would be determined more by local service providers through their curriculum development and commissioning groups than by the interpretation of centralised syllabuses. The function of accrediting bodies would be to ensure that any relevant standards were maintained in keeping with their own quality assurance mechanism. Extant practice would, therefore, evolve from the programme content. It would not be 'taught' as part of the programme but be developed through activities integral to the programme and would relate directly to client and consumer need.

Refined practice and enhanced understanding

It is within the practice area that the outcomes of this learning cycle should have their main impact. It would be by no means essential for the service provider already to be at the forefront of contemporary systems of delivery. Quite the opposite; while such areas may exist, they tend to be small scale and often function in isolation. Indeed, this may well be what has enabled such areas to progress, because of the degree of control and specificity they are able to bring to their service. It would be the intention of the programmes of education and training to capitalise upon such models and to increase the transferability of skills and knowledge across a broader field of services through an educational process that encourages and enables the sharing of information rather than compartmentalisation. The enhanced understanding of outcoming students must be supported by this concept if they are to benefit services as a whole.

One of the features of reorganisation of health and social services since the NHS and Community Care Act 1990 has been the advent of purchasing authorities fulfilling their role as commissioning agents for services. Mentally disordered offenders have become the focus for public attention since events involving Christopher Clunis and others. If a seamless service is the means by which to achieve an improved life-long service for individuals experiencing mental disorder who may be dangerous, it is the refinement of existing practice and the continuous evolution of levels of understanding that will provide a basis for measuring the value-for-money component that commissioning authorities can exercise. It would appear more appropriate, given the transient nature of the needs of the client group for health and social care, for organisations to act as a consortium and a focus for the purchasing of such services. Within that context, refined practice and enhanced knowledge could be achieved and verified across a range of statutory, private and voluntary providers.

The refinement of practice and the enhancement of understanding could relate as much to personal function within a plural service as to the application of methods and interventions with specific clients. Associated communication skills and care management techniques could feature highly in the various levels of the programme. The efficacy of joint and shared learning would be measured alongside individual learning outcomes.

Commissioners of services have an ideal opportunity to overcome the professional isolationism that contributed so significantly to the mismanagement of the care of Christopher Clunis. Brown (1994, p. 62) explains how employer-led training and education has radically challenged:

> the historical dominance of profession-determined education. Involvement of employers at a regional level in Training and Enterprise Councils is mirrored in specific programmes such as GTEC Diploma and ACCESS courses. Employers are increasingly being involved and integrated within the Diploma in Social Work as they are in health service training. In spite of the antipathy of the nursing profession to contribute to the development of competence based training it is clear, nonetheless, that 'competence' as promulgated by the National Council for Vocational Qualifications is the currency in which all future training programmes will have to be expressed. Shared learning is no exception.

Increased quality of individualised care

The emphasis throughout this chapter has been upon the integration of theory with practice and the measurement of educational outcomes in terms of their influence on individual client care. When refined practice and enhanced knowledge are demonstrated, it will be to the benefit of the organisation and the individual practitioner. It may well be that the organisation is able to offer new or refined services on the basis of that person's refined competence; the practitioner or care worker may be enabled to cross incremental thresholds by attaining qualifications. What is not always evident is how individual clients benefit from these advances.

By linking the learning cycle to the specific care programme of individual client(s), it becomes increasingly possible to measure the effect of the outcomes of education and training. The criteria for the judgement of loss or gain should be taken from aspects of the individual care plan and the quality development plan of the service. This would enable outcomes to be judged within the specificity of patient/client care. While the organisation may be set targets for efficiency and cost benefit, it needs to take a longer-term perspective regarding its investment in training and education. The advent of market economies in health and social care has led to a tendency for providers to think in a very short-term time frame that is dictated by the duration and nature of existing contracts. It is the very nature of needs associated with this client group, that is, they are long term and of high intensity, that makes them a high-cost care group. Any return on investments in education and training must be viewed within that time frame. An increased quality of individualised care need not carry an increased financial burden. The results of an employer-led system of education and training, based upon a consortium of interests, could be a more appropriate utilisation of human resources. This can best be measured with respect to individualised programmes of care rather than to a review of block contracts.

Summary

What is proposed within this chapter is a format and framework for the preparation of care staff and practitioners to work in services that are specifically targeted at the needs of individuals whose violent and/or aggressive behaviours represent special needs. It assumes that there is a commitment from any interested parties to accept their existing deficits and to invest in a service that will have an educational and operational philosophy compatible with creating learning opportunities for all consumers and staff. In a competitive environment, this is essential for all concerned. If an organisation is to survive, the rate of learning of its people must be equal to or greater than the rate of change in its environment, this environment including the social, economic and political influences that are affecting that organisation.

Where an organisation is providing services for a group of clients whose needs are as complex as those associated with people who have a mental illness or a developmental impairment, the rate of change in the environment is, indeed, rapid. Where this is further complicated by what are felt to be antisocial behaviours, the intensity of change in the environment can be as unpredictable as it is frequent. For these reasons, the education and training of staff to work with this client group must be a constituent, but central, part of the overall development of a learning organisation, driven by the needs of the client group.

Ultimately, people with a mental disorder who present as dangerous/violent have a right to excellent services that recognise their intrinsic human value and individuality and their need for skilled therapeutic intervention. This recognition must be reflected in the education of service providers.

References

Audit Commission (1986) *Making A Reality of Community Care*, HMSO, London.

Beacock C. (1994) A journey without end: creating a development strategy for staff in secure forensic settings. In Thompson A. and Mathias P. (eds) *Lyttle's Mental Health and Disorder*, London, Baillière Tindall.

Brown J. (1994) *The Hybrid Worker*, York, University of York.

Department of Health (1990) *Needs and Responses*, London, HMSO.

Department of Health (1993) *Services for People with Learning Disabilities and Challenging Behaviour or Mental Health Needs*, London, HMSO.

Department of Health and Home Office (1992) *Review of Health and Social Services for Mentally Impaired Offenders and Others Requiring Similar Services: Final Summary Report* (Reed Report), London, HMSO.

Department of Health and Special Hospitals Authority (1992) *Report of the Committee of Inquiry into Complaints about Ashworth Hospital* (Blom-Cooper Report), London, HMSO.

Department of Health and Social Security (1971) *Revised Report of the Working Party on Security in the NHS Psychiatric Hospitals* (Glancy Report), London, HMSO.

Department of Health and Social Security and Home Office (1974) *Interim Report of the Committee on Mentally Abnormal Offenders* (Butler Report), London, HMSO.

Goffman E. (1961) *Asylums: Essays on the Social Situation of Mental Patients and Other Inmates*, Doubleday, New York.

NE Thames and SE Thames RHAs (1994) *Report of the Inquiry into the Care and Treatment of Christopher Clunis* (Clunis Report), London, HMSO.

Royal College of Psychiatrists (1980) *Secure Facilities for Psychiatric Patients: A Comprehensive Policy*, London, Royal College of Psychiatrists.

Sheppard D. (1994) *Learning the Lessons: Mental Health Inquiry Reports Published in England and Wales Between 1969–1994 and their Recommendations for Improving Practice*, London, Zito Trust.

Tomlinson, B. (1992) *Report of the Inquiry into London's Health Service, Medical Education and Research*. Presented to the Secretaries of State for Health and Education by Sir Bernard Tomlinson, London, HMSO.

Tuxworth E. (1989) Competence-based education and training: background and origins. In Burke J. (ed.) *Competency Based Education and Training*, London, Falmer Press.

UKCC (1992) *Code of Professional Conduct*, London, UKCC.

UKCC (1994) *The Council's Standards for Education and Practice Following Registration*, London, UKCC.

10

THE ROLE OF THE MANAGER

John Turnbull

Introduction

Throughout this book, all the contributors have sought to emphasise three key points about violence and aggression that must be acknowledged before the problem can be managed successfully.

First, violence, or the fear of violence, is almost a daily hazard for many people working in public services. Some groups of staff, for example nurses, face the greatest risk of assault, particularly those working with people with mental health problems or learning disabilities (Health Services Advisory Committee 1987). It is unclear in what ways the closure of many of the long-stay hospitals for these groups of people is affecting this picture. Social workers are another vulnerable group of staff, particularly where their work is associated with administering child protection procedures. Increasingly, reports from general practitioners and teachers are highlighting the need to take more seriously the risks they face.

The second point is that whereas it is possible to isolate a particular 'trigger' for violent incidents, violence and aggression are dynamic processes in which it is impossible to identify a single underlying cause. Given the right circumstances, anyone is capable of becoming violent. This makes single solutions to the problem particularly difficult to find.

Finally, violence and aggression should be seen as an occupational rather than a clinical problem. Whereas it is true that many of the assaults on staff are perpetrated by people receiving treatment or care for behaviour that includes a lack of self-control or aggression, a significant number of assaults will be carried out by people who have no history of violence. These people could be distressed relatives or others who come into contact with services at times of stress. Some, for example, may be in pain or have recently been bereaved. The key point is that whereas staff are paid to deal with the public under very challenging circumstances, they are not paid to be hit or traumatised. To put it another way, staff are assaulted *because* they are at work (Greaves 1994). Therefore, the problem is an occupational one.

Many of the chapters in this book have described techniques and approaches that will help individual staff to cope better with potential or actual violence. But what of the role of managers? Managers are responsible for developing systems of work that enable the staff to work safely and to work towards achieving the aims of the organisation that employs them. Given the risk and extent of violence and aggression within services, it would appear that managers are not coping well with the problem. Therefore, this concluding chapter will clarify the manager's role by recommending approaches by which violence and aggression could be better managed. This will be achieved by presenting a framework through which the risk of violence to staff can be assessed and reduced. First, however, we need to clarify what management is for.

What is management for and how do you do it?

If we were asked about management and its purpose, most of us would begin by thinking about people we have been managed by in the past and describe it in terms of the personal characteristics of those managers. Likewise, much of the management literature has traditionally discussed management in terms of the individual style of managers, for example describing them as authoritarian, democratic or *laissez-faire*. On a day-to-day basis, it is important to us, of course, how our managers behave towards us. However, this is only one aspect of management. A focus on personality alone will tell us little about how violence and aggression might be better managed. Therefore, this chapter will concentrate more on the process of management rather than managers themselves.

So, what is management supposed to do? For as long as work has needed to be done by groups of people, there have been forces or processes influencing how the work has been carried out. Much of this is the area of responsibility of management. However, the systematic study of management is a relatively new phenomenon and is even more rare in connection with public services.

Despite this growing literature, a convenient definition of management remains elusive. Many writers have emphasised the controlling function of management; others see management as being synonymous with decision-making. Wille (1992) describes management as 'risking yourself in the mobilising of resources and relationships to add value to the enterprise' (p. 1). Handy (199 defines management as 'the missing X which makes resources equal output' (p. 320). From these descriptions, the purpose of management seems to be to ensure that a task or set of tasks is carried out efficiently and effectively. However, how to achieve this is a different matter.

Management has gone through a number of changes in the past two decades. The emphasis on decision-making and controlling that once existed was popular when organisations were seen as large machines in which workers made up the parts and were expected to react when the manager 'threw' a switch. Today organisations are seen more as a 'brain', capable of learning and adapting in what is a rapidly changing and complex world. The role of the manager in this scenario is much different. Here, he or she is seen as an enabler and leader, aiming to get the best out of each individual. Structures within such organisations reflect this as the traditional hierarchy is taken down and more responsibility is passed over to the employee. This is an important factor when thinking about managing violence. Although violent incidents will share particular characteristics, each one is unique. Therefore, staff will have to be prepared to adapt their skills to each situation. The manager's role is not to 'hand down' instructions but to set a framework within which the staff's own skills and creativity can be encouraged. So, what should this framework consist of?

Managing violence and aggression

Managing violence and aggression is, of course, not the central purpose of an organisation. Instead, it is a byproduct or unwanted consequence of the organisation's key activity. In health, for example, the purpose of a service is to improve the health of its local population by treating illness and helping individuals to keep well. Violence to the staff who are working towards these goals will threaten progress. For example, a demotivated and fearful staff will ultimately distance themselves from those whom they are trying to treat and care for unless they are supported. This will have negative consequences for the quality of care delivered. There will also be serious financial implications for the service, for example in terms of greater staff sickness and turnover, if violence is not managed.

Staff will often be reluctant to work in certain areas, and the service will begin to lose its reputation.

Clearly, violence and aggression pose significant risks to the efficiency and effectiveness of a service. There are several specific approaches that can be taken to manage the problem, which will be described shortly. However, it is important that we see these approaches within an overall framework as it is rare for one particular approach to be successful on its own. Therefore, a model that has been chosen for use in this chapter is one based on risk management.

Risks are nothing new to public services. For example, it is inevitable that the demand for services will outstrip the ability to supply and the decision to admit one person to a bed will mean that others have to wait, potentially leading to a worsening of their condition. One the other hand, developments in services and treatments would not have been achieved if someone had not been prepared to take calculated risks. However, as the National Health Service Executive (1993) has pointed out, the delivery of services to the public is increasingly becoming a risky business. Since the abolition of Crown Immunity in 1991, public services have become individually liable for their actions and the payment of compensation in the event of a mistake. Many services are also now functioning in the context of a managed market for services in which contracts could be placed with competitors if their performance failed to meet the set criteria. The contracting-out of services within the public sector can give rise to a feeling of not being in full control of services. Similarly, the public sector has witnessed considerably greater decentralisation of its services in recent years, along with a flattening of its management structure. Some would say that this has brought pressures for professional staff and others to work beyond their level of competence.

Traditional approaches to managing these risks have been unsystematic and reactive. In many cases, risk has been managed by denial, avoidance or claims that events such as violent incidents are unforeseeable and are, therefore, accidents. Interestingly, many staff still record incidents on 'accident forms', thus reinforcing this view. The experience of staff as well as the growing research literature on the nature of violence and its management have challenged this view, and there is a need to take a more proactive and systematic approach to the problem.

The nature of risk

The *Concise Oxford English Dictionary* defines risk simply as 'a hazard'. Given the choice, most of us would like to avoid the unpleasant consequences of our own or other people's actions. However, because we know that there are risks in practically every activity, we all become engaged in an almost unconscious risk management process each day. This process first involves us making a judgement about the likely positive and negative consequences of our actions. If the result is that we can foresee greater potential benefits than losses, we are likely to accept the risk. For example, we know that the incidence of crime in urban areas is higher than in rural communities. However, the advantages for us in terms of proximity to our place of work and accessibility to a range of shops and entertainment facilities usually means that we would opt for a city life.

However, risk management is not simply about weighing good consequences against bad. Harris *et al.* (1996) point out that there are two components to risk assessment:

1. The likelihood that actions will lead to positive or negative outcomes
2. The relative size or significance of those outcomes.

In their book on physical interventions, Harris and his colleagues go on to explain how these components interact (Table 10.1).

Some activities carry with them a high probability that something will go wrong, but we may still decide to accept the risks based on our judgement of their impact. For example, in Table 10.1, the sport of cave diving not only has a high probability of accidents happening, but also the consequences of these accidents are grave in terms of injury and death. The consequences of an aeroplane accident are just as serious, but, statistically speaking, we know that accidents are very infrequent. Some events have a high probability of loss occurring for the individual, as in the case of buying a National Lottery ticket. However, for most people, the loss is affordable and is considered to be of low impact. Finally, the chances of a mistake happening when following a simple recipe are low, as are the consequences if things do go wrong.

Table 10.1   Level of perceived risk of adverse outcomes

Consequences	High probability	Low probability
High impact	Cave diving	Air travel
Low impact	Buying a lottery ticket	Using a new recipe to make a cake

Before moving on, it should be remembered that inaction can be just as risky as action. For example, continuing to eat a high-fat diet, smoking and taking minimal exercise will increase the probability of heart disease. Therefore, risks are present in every aspect of our daily lives and cannot be avoided simply by doing nothing.

Managing risk in public services

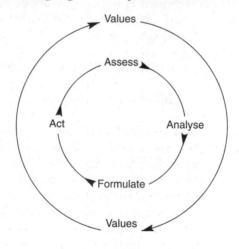

Partnership

Figure 10.1   Framework for managing risk

The same principles apply to risk management in public services as they do to individual decision-making. However, whereas individual risk management is largely an unconscious process, the manager has the responsibility to take a more systematic and overt approach. The remainder of this chapter will focus on a framework for risk management for violence and aggression, which is shown in Figure 10.1. This model is presented as a series of discrete steps. In reality, there is a great deal of overlap, but the sections that follow will set out important questions for the manager for each stage and provide examples of how these questions might be answered. The key questions can be found in Table 10.2.

Table 10.2   Key questions in the management of violence

Values	What does the organisation stand for?
	What are the beliefs and principles held by staff?
Assess	What are the sources of information?
	How can information collection be improved?
	Who should collect it?
Analyse	What is the potential for risk?
	What is its probable impact?
	What Is the financial cost of taking action/not taking action?
Formulate	What is the plan to minimise the risk?
	Is it compatible with the aims of the service?
	What will staff have to do differently?
Act	How will the plan be implemented?
	How will good practice be maintained?
	What are the criteria for success?

Step one: Values

Although this has been listed as a component of the risk management process, it should, in reality, underpin the entire process. The values held by staff within a service give the organisation its culture, which in turn lies behind many of the decisions taken by staff and managers. Implementing a new procedure, such as risk management, or maintaining an existing one must take account of the principles and beliefs held by people within an organisation. All procedures should be compatible with the values of the organisation.

Public service organisations such as health, social services and education usually have in common a set of values and principles underpinning their work. Put simply, these may be described as:

- A belief that each person is unique
- A belief that all people have equal value
- That services should act at all times in the best interests of the individual
- That services should do the least possible harm to the individual.

Translated into day-to-day activity, this means that the needs of each person will be assessed individually and have a plan of care, education or support that is as individualised as possible. However, as we know, there are many things that can get in the way of this, some of which are unique to public services. First of all, public services employ a range of professional staff who work within a framework of beliefs and principles provided by their separate codes of professional conduct. While this is important, the significant fact from the manager's point of view is that it is non-professional staff who will have the greatest amount of contact with service users. These staff have no code of conduct, and the manager is left with the dilemma of whether to develop a code for the entire service or introduce a separate one for non-professional staff. Commenting on this, Flynn (1995) believes that it would be impossible to supplant existing codes of conduct with one that is unique to the service. However, this should not deter the manager from seeking agreement over or reinforcing key principles to complement those already in existence.

A second problem facing many public service organisations is the fact that the users of the service often do not choose to use it and may not respond sympathetically to the altruistic motives of staff. Prisoners, for example, do not ask to be incarcerated. Victims of road traffic accidents have little choice but to use accident and emergency facilities, and children have no choice whether they receive education. This may affect the way in which the service user acts, which can, in turn, make it difficult for the staff to maintain their beliefs and principles. For example, a client with learning disabilities may need to interact more with others as a prerequisite to using community facilities and enjoying a better quality of life. He may resent the encouragement of staff and respond by biting and hitting out at staff. Avoiding the risk by doing nothing might seem the simplest option and would prevent injury, but what would be the effect for the individual in the long term? Managers will have a key role to play here in helping staff to cope with this and to maintain their motivation.

A third problem is that the person who uses the service is not the only person to whom staff and managers are accountable, especially following many of the reforms in public services in recent years. Government, commissioners of services, colleagues, professional staff in the organisation and the wider public, as tax payers, could all be regarded as 'customers'. Such a range of people inevitably causes tension, which must be managed sensitively and could, at times, compromise the principle of working in the best interests of the individual. For example, commissioners of services may apply pressure for community nursing staff to increase their caseloads. Nurses may feel that this will compromise the quality of support they will be able to provide. It could be that this could provoke frustrations among clients and staff alike. Requests for separate funding for personal alarms may present managers with choices of whether to finance them from existing resources and cut a service to the client or turn down the request. More recently, we have seen teachers in one school threatening strike action over a minority of disruptive and violent pupils. One of the key issues for the headteacher and governors here was whether to allow the actions of a minority of children to affect the education of the majority.

There are no simple answers to questions such as these. No doubt, violence could be managed more effectively by providing security guards to accompany community nurses or by erecting physical barriers between staff and the public, but few people would agree that this represents a way forward. If the essential values that distinguish public services are compromised, all of us will suffer.

Step two: Assess

This step in the risk management process is concerned with identifying the sources of information within a service that will be useful, how this information should be collected, who should collect it and how the process could be improved. At the outset, the manager will want to obtain as much information as possible prior to developing an approach to managing violence and aggression. However, it might be worthwhile bearing in mind that, whereas there is no limit to the amount of information that could be gathered, there is a limit to the amount of time that staff will tolerate before action is taken. In other words, the manager must take a pragmatic view.

Many people might believe that there is a shortage of information in services. In reality, services are a rich source of data. Thus any problems with information are usually to do with its interpretation rather than its generation. There has been an encouraging trend in recent years within services to employ staff in positions such as 'information officer'. Regrettably, these positions have a low status within organisations, and there is often confusion over whether occupants are responsible for getting or giving information or both. If services have developed information strategies or policies, this will help initiatives to manage violence and aggression. If not, a good start can be made by designating a manager in the organisation with responsibility for gathering, interpreting and communicating information in this important area.

Put simply, information available within services can be divided into two categories, 'formal' and 'informal'. The types of information that will fall into these categories are shown in Table 10.3, although this is by no means an exhaustive list. Both types are equally important, but the key sources of information required to manage violence are records of incidents themselves.

Table 10.3 Formal and informal sources of information

Formal	Informal
Incident report forms	Discussions with individuals
Care plans	or groups of staff
Finance reports	Focus groups
Complaints forms	Observation – 'management by
Sickness/absence records	wandering about'
Staff training records	Discussions with clients/patients
Staffing records –	and representative
use of agency	groups
staff/skill mix	Local/national newspapers

Having said this, records of violent incidents are notoriously unreliable in that they rarely match the actual levels of violence and aggression within services. Research by Lion *et al.* (1981), for example, estimated that official records of incidents should be multiplied five times in order to arrive at a more accurate figure. As well as the quantity of information, the manager must also address issues relating to its quality and ask whether the information requested on forms helps or hinders the process of risk management. From the victim's point of view, incident forms are important in any subsequent claim that he or she wishes to make against the employer. Managers will also require information that could help them to defend such an action, and details about the specific actions of the member of staff before and during the incident will be important. However, a balance needs to be found between getting the detail and getting the compliance of staff. Poyner and Warne (1986, para. 55) suggest the following categories as a minimum requirement for recording forms:

■ The characteristics of the assailant(s)
■ Information about the victim (employee)
■ A brief account of what happened before and during the incident
■ Details of the situation in which the incident took place
■ Details of the outcome (injury, action taken and so on).

To increase compliance, it is also worth considering whether forms could be designed to prevent the victim having to repeat information. For example, providing boxes to 'tick' for standard information could save time and possibly further distress for victims when recalling events. A helpful suggestion is provided by Howells and Hollin (1989), who describe a form used in a young offenders' centre. Under the general heading of describing the incident, this section is divided into 'Antecedents', 'Behaviour' and 'Consequences'. Importantly, this links the incident to any treatment or care being provided for certain clients and could be useful in identifying any consistent trigger factors or setting conditions for violence. Staff compliance could be increased as this is the type of information that they would wish to gather as part of the process of caring for the client.

Even if the culture within an organisation encourages the recording of incidents, the manager needs to be aware that records will still differ from the actual level of violence or threats of violence to which staff will be subjected. For this reason, it is useful to initiate periodic surveys of incidents. For example, for 1 day every 6 months, staff could be asked to use a simple and anonymous system of recording. Turnbull (1992) used a portable golf score counter, divided into categories according to the 'hole' number, with which staff recorded incidents of different types of challenging behaviour. These categories could easily be adapted to include verbal abuse, threats, intimidating gestures or actual assault and so on.

Care plans are another source of information that can be used to supplement incident forms. Whereas the organisation might not have time to aggregate information from all of these records, a retrospective sample of notes on people who have been involved in incidents might identify common factors.

Similarly, records of complaints made by clients, relatives or visitors can provide valuable insight into factors that could lead to incidents in the future. The nature of complaints means that they are either quite specific, such as a client complaining that he or she is not provided with pain relief in sufficient time when the staff are asked, or more general, such as a visitor who complains that the staff seem too busy to find time for their relative. In terms of violence and aggression, both should be taken as early warning signs of potential trouble.

There is no doubt that violence and aggression towards staff have a financial consequence for the organisation. Having said this, it is difficult to estimate precisely the cost of violence to the organisation, although this should appear as a category at the assessment stage in order to draw attention to the more positive potential use of these resources. Managers will need this information if they are making a case for investment in preventive strategies such as training. Few studies have addressed this issue specifically, and these have usually taken place in American settings that are not directly comparable to those of the United Kingdom. Nevertheless, Hill and Spreat (1987) calculated the cost per staff injury to be $2070. This is based on 40 successful claims by individuals in 1 year against a single employer in a 284-bedded hospital for people with learning disabilities. The annual cost, therefore, approximates to $80,000. Lanza and Milner (1989) studied the resources needed in terms of staff time spent in managing the consequences of incidents over a 4-month period in a hospital facility in the United States. They estimated the annual cost to the organisation to be $38,000. This study took no account of claims for compensation.

Where estimates have been made in the United Kingdom, it is usually in connection with stress across all sectors of business and commerce. Mathews (1992) estimated the cost of stress in absenteeism alone to be £1.3 billion. We know that managing violence on a day-to-day basis is stressful for staff, but it is impossible to estimate what proportion of this amount can be accounted for by violence alone. However, at a local level, managers could monitor sickness and absences in order to correlate this with information on levels of violence from incident forms. Furthermore, training records of staff could be used in a similar way. There is growing evidence that training in managing violence reduces the levels experienced by staff (Gertz 1980). Knowledge of who has skills in managing violence could also play a significant role when decisions over the deployment of staff need to be taken.

Staffing records will also be a source of information that managers will wish to monitor and correlate with recorded incidents. Research cannot establish a firm link between levels of violence and the numbers or qualifications of staff (Way *et al.* 1992). This does not mean that the issue can be discounted, and what seems to be more important is the way in which staff interact with clients and the way in which the staff behave as a team. Therefore, the use of staff unfamiliar to each other, such as agency staff, may affect their confidence in each other and their ability to work towards preventing incidents and managing them in a co-ordinated way if they occur.

From an informal point of view, the manager needs to take any opportunity of discussing key issues with staff, those who use the service or their representatives, such as Community Health Councils and even relatives when appropriate. The objective here is to gain information on how the service looks and feels like to those people. These opportunities might present themselves during pre-arranged or regular meetings, but there is also little substitute for 'walking the patch' or, to use another expression, 'managing by wandering about'. Alternatively, specific focus groups could be arranged to encourage views to be expressed, and although the manager may take responsibility for initiating these events, he or she should consider whether his or her presence at the event would encourage or discourage information to be shared. Outside facilitators can be useful in resolving this dilemma.

Finally, as management becomes more outward looking, managers need to acknowledge the context in which they are providing a service. This means being aware of the potential impact of changes in society on the service they offer. It is generally felt that people in society now have higher expectations of public services, want the freedom to pursue more individualistic lifestyles and possess more information about issues affecting their quality of life. While this is a positive development, it could also bring with it the potential for conflict if services cannot live up to expectations. A more negative feature of modern society is the reported increase in crime and alcohol and drug misuse. While the manager cannot be held responsible for putting this right, these changes may be reflected in the mix of cases referred to services.

To conclude this section on assessment, it is also worthwhile reflecting on who should be involved in gathering information. There are advantages in managers and staff in each service collecting the necessary information and looking for ways of improving the process because of their detailed knowledge of the service. On the other hand, a case could be made for involving outsiders because of the need for a more objective viewpoint. One way of doing this is through the growing number of risk management consultants, although their experience in the public sector is variable. The Health and Safety Executive or the police could also offer assistance in specialised areas. However, one of the most productive ways would be to invite managers and staff from a neighbouring or similar service. This could combine the need for objectivity as well as a knowledge of the issues. It could also encourage greater involvement from front-line staff because of the credibility that these consultants would bring to the process.

Step three: Analyse

The previous section focused on the information needed to manage violence more successfully and suggested improvements in its quality and quantity. This section follows on by looking at the ways in which this information can be organised in order to evaluate the potential for violence to staff within public services.

Whereas some possibilities in life can be described in terms of percentages, this is not the case in relation to violence. We have already seen from other chapters that violence is a product of an interaction between a variety of factors. With so many possibilities, assigning a numerical value to the risk is difficult. However, some distinction can be made through a process of what is known as social validity (Kazdin and Matson 1981). This means asking people, in this case managers and staff, to use a combination of their experience and intuition, supported by evidence, to rate a particular situation according to severity of risk. In practice, this could mean asking people to rate a situation as either low, medium or high risk.

It is impossible to consider here every combination of events that could lead to violence. For one thing, services will differ greatly from each other, but some core principles and a framework for analysis will be set out.

In estimating risk, it is useful to think of violence occurring at the intersection of three factors consisting of the assailant, the victim and the situation. This is shown in Figure 10.2. Although we need information on all three elements, risk cannot be assessed without applying a judgement on how we think they will interact. For example, first consider the example of a road traffic accident for which we need two drivers, one of whom is late for an appointment. Would our judgement of risk be different if it was a Monday or Sunday morning? What would we think if it was a foggy day in the middle of a major city?

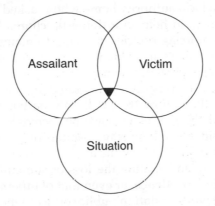

Figure 10.2   Key elements of a violent confrontation

Now consider the following example in terms of the risk of violence to staff. A local authority children's home provides a service for children, some of whom have a history of violent and aggressive outbursts towards staff. The staff in the home prepare individual plans for the support of each child, which are updated twice a day to include any changes in the child's circumstances, mood and so on. This is a positive feature that might be rated low in terms of risk of violence. However, if an assessment of other working practices of the staff reveals that there are few opportunities for staff to communicate with each other and there is a lack of time for staff to spend reading records, the rating would probably be of a higher level of risk.

From this, we can see the significance of working practices and routines in creating situations in which violence could occur. Although individual judgements will need to be applied to each situation, it is possible to identify broad categories of situational factors that will help in estimating risk.

Cessation or anticipated cessation of a positive experience

This is a factor that many researchers and writers on violence consider to be the most significant precipitator of violence and aggression. In an investigation by Sheridan *et al.* (1990) for example, this category came highest on the list of causes of violence. There are several examples we could think of in connection with this, such as the child in a local authority home who is asked to stop watching television in order to help in a domestic chore. Another example could be staff enforcing policies or trying to maintain routines that compromise someone's individual freedom. A ban on smoking in an accident and emergency department or general practitioner's waiting room will probably be tolerated by the majority of the public because they know they will only be temporarily inconvenienced. Would the risk of violence be increased if this ban were extended to residents of long-stay hospitals or nursing homes?

We should also think here of the anxiety or fear that can be generated in people by anticipating the loss of something such as their own health or independence, or even that of others. There are many instances in the work of staff in public services when people need to be helped to adjust or when bad news needs to be broken. This presents a risk if it is not managed appropriately.

Denial/cancellation of an anticipated event

We will all be aware of the psychological as well as practical preparation that is carried out in anticipation of some event, whether this is a holiday, a meal for relatives and friends or even a meeting with a bank manager. This applies equally, if not more, to public services, and any interruption or cancellation of the event causes disappointment and even anger. Therefore, managers need to be aware of the potential impact of cancelled appointments with therapists or consultants or case conferences that need to be re-arranged. Other examples that would fit into this category include denial of access to information or an explanation if it were anticipated by the individual. For example, a social worker may have come across information concerning a person's claim for benefits that could be communicated to that person, but he or she may decide that this could be held back until the picture becomes clearer.

This category would also include the blunting of expectations that often occurs between the public and the services they use. As mentioned earlier, the public have raised their expectations of services, and good practice would now dictate that the organisation should set out as clearly as possible what type of service the public is entitled to receive. When judging the potential risk to staff, the manager would clearly have an interest in looking at this aspect of working practice.

Failure to prevent an unpleasant event

It would be an impossible task for public services to prevent every negative event that happened to an individual during his or her contact with the service. However, services can take action to ensure that these events are not prolonged or repeated. For example, a person who has asked for his medication to be changed because of its unpleasant side-effects or someone whose pain is not controlled is likely to become more aroused if the matter is not dealt with satisfactorily. In medium- or long-term care settings, a resident may complain of the verbal abuse or threats from a fellow resident. The risk of the resident taking matters into his own hands is increased if the issue is ignored, delayed or denied.

Included in this category is waiting. Again, this is a factor considered by writers on the subject (Poyner and Warne 1986) to be significant in increasing the risk of violence. There are obvious examples of this, such as people waiting to see a consultant or a benefits officer. However, we should also consider the point of view of people who are in medium- or long-term care settings such as hospitals, residential or nursing homes in which a lack of activity and stimulation have been identified as contributors to violence (Weaver *et al.* 1978). Under these conditions, the client could be regarded as simply waiting for the next event, for example a meal or a visit from a relative.

Time of day and week

The time of day and time of the week can create circumstances in which the risk of violence is increased. For example, although people can now get access to alcohol at almost any time during the day, its effects are more likely to increase risk after 11 p.m. when pubs and bars are closing. This is well known to accident and emergency departments in hospitals, but it could also be a factor in other settings where people may try to visit their friends and relatives. Similarly, weekends are times when people will take the opportunity to relax, but this could result in some becoming disinhibited.

In residential settings, some research indicates that night times present a relatively low risk of violence, simply because most people are asleep. On the other hand, for some residents, night times can be occasions when people ruminate on problems.

For staff who make visits to clients during the night, for example general practitioners, social workers or even ambulance staff, the darkness can provide cover for those intent on stealing drugs or equipment.

Isolation of staff

Following on from this, services are increasingly being delivered in community settings in people's homes. Whereas many, including the client, would see this as a positive move, managers must be aware that this prevents staff accessing the type of help that can be mobilised in a residential setting. Working in people's homes also presents opportunities for more serious and frightening examples of violence, such as hostage-taking. There has been a great deal written about the sort of action that can be taken to minimise risk, which will be discussed in the next section. However, managers should also make judgements about other times when a member of staff is isolated and more vulnerable, for example when travelling between home and the workplace. The possibility that a potential assailant could target a member of staff in his or her home should also be taken into account.

Step four: Formulation

In the next stage of the risk management process, the manager has the responsibility for devising approaches that will minimise the risk of violence to staff or, in some cases, accepting the risk. The manager should now have a desk full of information, including evaluations of the different levels of risk posed by certain circumstances. It would be rare, however, for any manager to be able to resource and implement all the ideas that he or she has about managing those risks. Managers have difficult decisions to make, which need to take into account the following questions:

- What approaches can I take?
- Are they compatible with the values of the service?
- Do I have any information about their effectiveness?
- How differently will staff be expected to act?
- How long will it take to make changes?

Cost will be a major factor in implementing change and needs to be weighed against the likely reduction in risk. For example, it may be a good idea to change shift patterns to enable staff to have a longer handover time to communicate key information about clients. Such a change might result in a cost to the service of hundreds of thousands of pounds. An alternative might be to seek changes to shifts only in areas where incidents are more numerous. Alternatively, the introduction of handover or communication books might offer the right opportunity for staff to convey messages.

Time is another factor that must be taken into account. If the eventual aim is to develop better teamwork among staff in order that they can respond better to incidents, this will require investment in both team-building sessions and training as well as a reduction in the use of agency staff. This will increase costs, for which there will be no immediate benefit.

We can see from this that the manager needs to be practical and patient. He or she also needs to think flexibly enough to prioritise from a range of options. Solutions to the problem of violence need to be unique to the particular service. However, the following areas may provide useful information that may be used in formulating appropriate responses.

Improved interaction with clients

Public services are essentially human services in which the aims can only be achieved through interaction between those giving and those using the service. In looking for potential risk management approaches, interaction is a useful place to start. On the rare occasions when assailants have been asked what would have prevented them hitting out at staff, they have invariably mentioned better communication (Sheridan *et al.* 1990).

Authors such as Kagan *et al.* (1989) have written extensively on how to improve the quality of interaction of professional staff. In Chapter 6 on de-escalation, Paterson and Leadbetter have also pointed to patterns of interaction that minimise the risk of incidents becoming more serious. From the manager's point of view, the key areas for improvement would be:

- The availability of staff to interact
- The level and clarity of information given to clients.

It does not matter how skilled a communicator a member of staff happens to be, if he or she is not available to interact with clients, risk cannot be managed or prevented. In residential services, where levels of interaction have been measured, the results show extremely poor levels of staff-initiated contact with clients (Felce *et al.* 1991). Even when clients are capable of initiating contact by seeking out staff, they will be reluctant to do so if the staff always look preoccupied. There is a clear need, therefore, to assess workload and examine working practices in order to create the setting conditions for interaction to take place. Making time for clients is also a measure that is compatible with the aims and values of the service.

In community settings, availability is also an issue, but the emphasis will be on the availability of information for clients. As mentioned earlier, not knowing about something can result in higher arousal levels. Community staff should take every opportunity to clarify roles and expectations and give information where possible in advance of meetings and visits.

Communication between staff

The lack of communication between staff has been highlighted in the literature as being a major cause of clients being awarded damages against services (Kroll and McKenzie 1983). It has also been a prominent criticism in many of the official inquiries in recent years. At a service level, the manager needs to create opportunities for better communication, and some ideas have already been set out here to achieve this. However, in some services, communication between staff works perfectly well in that information is passed through what is known as 'the grapevine'. For example, certain clients who have been violent in the past can develop a reputation that is usually exaggerated or distorted. This leads to what some have called 'the incubation of fear' and not only creates negative expectations among staff, but also increases the risk of violence.

Managers need to be aware of this and take appropriate action. It may be a useful strategy for assessments carried out on some individuals to have a separate assessment of their capacity for violence, perhaps to include specific and known trigger factors for incidents. Although this could lead to accusations of labelling, this will have the beneficial effect of clarifying for staff the actual level of risk they may face and provide the basis for prevention strategies.

Training and education

Paterson and Leadbetter have already discussed the need to match the level of training in services to the level of perceived risk (Chapter 6). This ensures that resources are used efficiently and effectively. Although research in this area is sparse, there is some evidence to suggest that training can reduce incidents, but, even if this is true, its principal function is to reduce rather than eliminate risk entirely.

As well as specific training in approaches such as de-escalation and physical intervention, managers should also consider adopting similar approaches to fire training in the case of violent incidents. Such 'incident drills' can be useful in reducing arousal levels in staff, thus leading to clearer thinking and more confident action. Such procedures will also be useful in developing teamwork.

Helping isolated staff

For several years, there have existed a number of publications that address the specific needs of community staff in relation to minimising their risk of assault (Department of Health and Social

Security 1988). Despite their existence, it is disappointing to note that many services have failed to implement these strategies. It is also worrying, although not surprising, that in a recent report (Royal College of Nursing 1994) that asked staff about their greatest fear about working in the community, the response was working alone or working during the hours of darkness.

Good working practice in community settings would dictate that the following guidelines be followed as a minimum requirement:

- Make sure that the receptionist/secretary at your base has full details of your movements for the day.
- If you are concerned about the risk from a particular client, arrange for someone to telephone you during the visit on either a mobile or the client's telephone. The caller can then be reassured or alerted.
- If there is no response, implement a pre-arranged plan that may include telephoning the police.
- Carry the minimum amount of equipment, for example mobile telephones or medication, and let the public know through the local press in order to deter potential attackers.
- Do not wear uniform if you think that this will attract unwanted attention.
- If the client you visit has a dog, ask him to lock it in another room before you enter the house.

The manager's concern about isolated staff should not be confined to when they are on duty. Many staff, for example from hospitals, will walk home or travel on public transport in their uniforms, which can make them a target. Managers should consider, if applicable, providing and encouraging the use of a changing area in the hospital.

Special equipment and security devices

There have been no special studies of the effectiveness of special equipment in reducing levels of risk of violence to staff. Mobile telephones, as we have seen from the previous discussion, can be a valuable means of obtaining help if necessary. However, they can also be a target for thieves. From anecdotal evidence, personal alarms can be useful in summoning help in residential or day service settings but have little use in the community. Some people report that an alarm has prevented further attack, whereas others have reported the opposite, perhaps because the assailant was encouraged by this apparent display of fear.

The tragic incident witnessed in 1996 in Dunblane and the murder of headteacher Phillip Lawrence have shown how vulnerable staff and children can be when there is open access to premises. The increase in physical security measures taken since this time in schools and other public buildings is a welcome sight, even if this is at the expense of some inconvenience to all of us.

Step five: Act

The successful implementation of a strategy to manage violence relies upon the same good management practice needed to manage any other area of change. Implied throughout this chapter and illustrated in Figure 10.1 is the need for any approach to be developed in partnership with those whom it is going to affect. This obviously includes staff within a service and their professional or representative organisations. It also includes those who are commissioning services. They should be just as interested in raising standards of care and managing risk, and, if resources are required, it will be an advantage if they have been aware of plans from the beginning. Seldom, if at all, do managers consider involving people who use the service. This could provide opportunities to gain information on their experiences of interaction with staff. If any of them have experienced being restrained or have been calmed by the actions of staff, their views will be a source of valuable feedback. There is increasingly a willingness to involve the public in broad discussions about how health and social services can better solve their problems. We may be a long way off discussing risk management with them, but preparing for such an event might be worthwhile.

There is no space here to discuss the different ways in which change can be managed in organisations. However, an essential part of success rests with managers demonstrating their commitment to making the workplace safer. The prime indicator of this commitment is often seen as the service's policy on violence and aggression. Despite the legal requirements to safeguard the workforce, many services either do not yet have a policy on violence or have one that is of such poor quality as to be useless (Norris 1990). Frequently, and to illustrate the point made above, managers devise policies alone that take little account of what actually happens in practice. It is not surprising that staff fail to implement their guidelines.

Carol Kedward, writing about her research in this area in Norris (1990) sets out a minimum requirement for the topic areas that should appear in a policy document:

- A definition of violence
- A statement of responsibility on the part of the authority
- Some account of the incidence of violence and threats
- A commitment to appropriate training for all staff groups
- Preventive measures
- Warning signs
- Methods of handling violence
- Proper recording methods
- Clear instructions to line managers
- Availability of counselling help/team support
- Availability of financial help and entitlement
- Liaison with appropriate Trade Unions.

(Norris 1990, p. 99)

Services might want to add to this list the framework through which risk will be assessed and managed. It should also be remembered that policy documents exist to give a basic framework and, once produced, should be revised in the light of the organisation's experience and increasing confidence. For example, it would be useful to add a section committing the organisation to produce an annual risk prevention plan. Here, the service could set out the specific steps that will be taken in the coming 12 months to maintain a safe working environment. This plan could also include an evaluation of the success of the previous 12 months.

Conclusion

To briefly conclude this chapter, we have seen how a risk management framework can help the manager to identify key factors within the service and the practice of staff that can affect the level of risk to employees. This consists of gaining information, improving it if necessary and analysing it in order to make judgements about the potential risk and the financial consequences of inaction. This should lead to a plan that needs to be achievable and compatible with the values of the organisation. Finally, the implementation of

this plan must be carried out in partnership with the key stake-
holders in the organisation.

Ultimately, managing risk successfully helps the manager to
achieve the central task of improving the effectiveness and efficiency of the organisation. If carried out correctly, the values held by
the staff within the service will also be strengthened.

References

Department of Health and Social Security (1988) *Violence to Staff. Report of
the DHSS Advisory Committee on Violence to Staff,* London, HMSO.
Felce D., Repp A., Thomas M. *et al.* (1991) The relationship of staff:client
ratios, interactions and residential placement, *Research in Developmental
Disabilities,* **12**: 315–31.
Flynn N. (1995) *Public Sector Management,* 2nd edn, London, Harvester
Wheatsheaf.
Gertz B. (1980) Training for prevention of assaultive behaviour in a psychi-
atric setting, *Hospital and Community Psychiatry,* **31**: 628–30.
Greaves A. (1994) Organisational approaches to the prevention and
management of violence. In Whykes T. (ed.) *Violence and Health Care
Professionals,* London, Chapman & Hall.
Handy C. (1993) *Understanding Organisations,* 4th edn, Harmondsworth,
Penguin.
Harris J., Allen D., Cornick M. *et al.* (1996) *Physical Interventions. A Policy
Framework,* Kidderminster, British Institute of Learning Disabilities.
Health Services Advisory Committee (1987) *Violence to Staff in the Health
Service,* London, HMSO.
Hill J. and Spreat S. (1987) Staff injury rates associated with the implemen-
tation of contingent restraint, *Mental Retardation,* **25**(3): 141–3.
Howells K. and Hollin C.R. (eds) (1989) *Clinical Approaches to Violence,*
Chichester, John Wiley & Sons.
Kagan A.E., Evans J. and Kay B. (1989) *A Manual of Interpersonal Skills for
Nurses,* London, Harper Row.
Kazdin A.E. and Matson J.L. (1981) Social validation in mental retardation,
Applied Research in Mental Retardation, **2**: 39–53.
Kroll J. and McKenzie T.B. (1983) When psychiatrists are liable: risk
management and violent patients, *Hospital and Community Psychiatry,*
34(1): 29–37.
Lanza M. and Milner J. (1989) The dollar cost of patient assault, *Hospital and
Community Psychiatry,* **40**(12): 1227–9.
Lion J.R., Snyder W. and Merrill G.L. (1981) Under-reporting of assaults on
staff in a state hospital, *Hospital and Community Psychiatry,* **32**: 497–8.
Mathews L. (1992) Beating the office bully, *Industrial Society Briefing Plus,*
December: 4–5.
National Health Service Executive (1993) *Risk Management in the NHS,*
London, NHSE.

Norris D. (1990) *Violence against Social Workers. The Implications for Practice*, London, Jessica Kingsley.

Poyner B. and Warne C. (1986) *Violence to Staff. A Basis for Assessment and Prevention*, London, Health and Safety Executive.

Royal College of Nursing (1994) *Violence and Community Nursing Staff*, London, RCN.

Sheridan M., Henrion R., Robinson L. *et al.* (1990) Precipitants of violence in a psychiatric inpatient setting, *Hospital and Community Psychiatry*, **41**(7): 776–80.

Turnbull J. (1992) Quality of care for people with mental handicap and challenging behaviour. An evaluation of the impact of staff training in goal attainment scaling and behavioural procedures, unpublished Master's thesis, University of St Andrews, Fife.

Way B., Braff J., Hafemeister J. and Banks S. (1992) The relationship between patient–staff ratio and reported patient incidents, *Hospital and Community Psychiatry*, **43**(4): 361–5.

Weaver S.M., Broome A.K. and Bernard J.B. (1978) Some patterns of disturbed behaviour in a closed ward environment, *Journal of Advanced Nursing*, **3**: 251–63.

Wille E. (1992) *Quality: Achieving Excellence*, London, Century Business.

INDEX